Body and Mind in Motion

Body and Mind in Motion
Dance and Neuroscience in Conversation

Glenna Batson
with
Margaret Wilson

intellect Bristol, UK / Chicago, USA

First published in the UK in 2014 by
Intellect, The Mill, Parnall Road, Fishponds, Bristol, BS16 3JG, UK

First published in the USA in 2014 by
Intellect, The University of Chicago Press, 1427 E. 60th Street,
Chicago, IL 60637, USA

A catalogue record for this book is available from the
British Library.

Cover image: Courtesy of J Harper
Cover designer: Stephanie Sarlos
Copy-editor: Paul Nash
Production manager: Tim Mitchell
Typesetting: Contentra Technologies

Print ISBN: 978-1-78320-179-2
ePDF ISBN: 978-1-78320-236-2
ePUB ISBN: 978-1-78320-237-9

Printed and bound by TJ International, UK

To all my movement teachers whose aesthetic reached me ... who helped
me think, move, endure.

There is a straight ladder from the atom to the grain of sand, and the only
real mystery in physics is the missing rung. Below it, particle physics,
above it, classical physics, but in between, metaphysics. All the
mystery in life turns out to be this same mystery, the join
between things which are distinct and yet continuous,
body and mind, freewill and causality,
living cells and life itself.'

Tom Stoppard, *Hapgood,* Act I, Scene 5, 1988

Contents

Acknowledgments

This book is my gift to dance artists, educators and scholars – those just starting out and hopefully veterans as well. It is my way of paying homage to mentors who helped me find a living vocabulary – moving and spoken. To all these mentors in dance, science and somatic studies, I owe an enormous debt. My life would not be the same without an alchemical mix of treasured resources, ranging from teachers to books, students and praxis. Many in this pantheon are still working and continuing to inspire me to teach and mentor others. In my commitment to carry forward dance, Somatics and science, writing a book seems like a modest way to contribute to this legacy and pay it forward.

I carry the deepest appreciation for the generative power of dance. Many times during the writing of this book, I'd find myself stymied. I'd need a *mot juste*, a way of clarifying a concept or a route out of a chapter's organizational quagmire. I'd stop working and go to the studio. There, I'd dance out the answers. Nothing direct, mind you. The 'answers' unleashed themselves as my brittle body tensions gave way to gestural flow. I'd toss my mental confusion about in playful improvisation. This 'no-place-space' of body expressiveness would open portals of understanding that no amount of mental machinations could possibly have engineered. Movement provided the deepest intellectual satisfaction I could have ever imagined – as mover, as witness and ultimately, as scholar.

I bow low to a number of past dance teachers. Their combined inspiration, courage and commitment to living through the body brought logic to my life. These include Molly Lynn, Betty Jones, Judy van Zile, Erick Hawkins, Nadine Ravene, Bella Lewitsky, Marcia Sakamoto, Walter Nicks, Robert Ellis Dunn, Judith Lesch, Krishna Rao, Nancy Stark-Smith and Adriana Miller. The list could actually go on and on. I also could add a host of guest artists who set me on fire.

I also owe thanks to my many teachers in somatic education who continue to inspire me to teach others. First and foremost, I thank Irene Dowd, whose belief in my budding abilities as an educator, along with her unending patience and crystalline rigor, allowed me to set boldly forth on the path of movement education. From 1977, under Irene's tutelage, I gained an extraordinary view of the *all* that we were investigating. Our work together allowed me to access dynamic bodily processes that gave rise to embodied coordination in action. With her guidance, I honed my visual acuity through the practice of Ideokinesis. Irene's clarity of vision left me with an enduring appreciation of movement as both an art and a science.

Thanks also go to Bruce and Martha Fertman, my first teachers in the Alexander Technique. They transmitted an amazing body of knowledge to me with poetic reverence. What patience and support they offered as I struggled to find my way back to my Self. I have stayed the course in this work since enrolling in their certification program in 1983. Today, I remain part of a world community of Alexander Technique teachers. My love for this work continues to deepen from the early seeds that they sowed.

I also continue to grow and learn within other somatic disciplines. I thank my Continuum movement teacher, Rebecca Lawson, who channels this work so beautifully. Each *dive* into the perceptual ocean opens a portal of embodiment truth. To Susan Harper, somatic sage, I offer heartfelt appreciation for modeling the *teacher-vessel* – one who holds the learning for so many while embodying all the teachings.

I also owe thanks to Sylvie Fortin, who saw my early teaching as holding promise for an integrative approach to somatically informed dance education: in the early 1990s, Sylvie spent a summer studying my teaching at the American Dance Festival (ADF) while pursuing her doctoral degree. At the time, I believed I was, in fact, carving out a novel approach, but lacked a framework to explain it. Sylvie went on to spearhead her own brand of scholarship in the role of Somatics as empowering and informing dance teaching.

Thanks also go to my mentor, colleague and friend, Martha Myers. Martha was a pioneer, advocate and visionary from the inception of the interpenetrated fields of dance science and Somatics. Without Martha, the confluence between dance science and Somatics would be impoverished, indeed. Martha invited me teach at the ADF in 1986. I spent more than a quarter of a century teaching there. The ADF provided a laboratory to test my ideas, gain practical and theoretical grounding, and learn from the incredible body of dancers who attend each summer. I also thank Donna Faye Birchfield, who hired me to teach in the Hollins/ADF Masters in Fine Arts program from 2006, and to Jeffery Bullock, who continues to head this program, in keeping me on board through – and because of – fluxus.

I owe thanks to Dr. Emma Redding, Edel Quin, Sarah Irvine, Ashley McGill and all the wonderful staff and students of the Masters in Dance Science program at Trinity Laban Conservatoire of Music and Dance who worked alongside me during my Fulbright residency in 2009: I continue to lecture in this program and to collaborate with wonderful teachers there.

In writing this book, I needed a collaborator to keep my motivation high and my vision clear. I invited Dr. Margaret Wilson from the Department of Theatre and Dance at the University of Wyoming to join me. I chose Margaret as my co-pilot because I needed a writing companion who is an active dancer – someone immersed in movement as the primary source material for embodied knowledge. Further, Margaret is a 'vertical dancer,' spending much of her dance time hanging from rocks in Wyoming and collaborating with other aerial dancers all over the world. I also needed someone who could cross disciplines and fully embrace phenomenological embodiment. Margaret brought a great deal to the table in dance, Somatics and dance science. Her experience made her a perfect choice. Over the last four years, we have mutually mentored one another in our research on dancers' balance, co-creating on a number of levels that have made the rigors of research downright fun. Together, we scouted unnamed territory and laid down tracks in pursuit of a nascent discourse.

This book wouldn't read with any degree of fluidity without the help of my beloved friend and superlative editor, Margaret (Peggy) Willig Crane. She is nothing short of a Renaissance woman: crossover singer, poet, documentary filmmaker, public relations expert…in short, her editorial mastery springs from a cornucopia of abundant creativity that brings musicality and visual brilliance to the written word.

I also thank Tim Mitchell, Production Manager and all the editorial staff of Intellect Press for their courteous and expert assistance throughout this whole publishing process.

Finally, I thank my parents, Clifton Batson and Linda Verrill Batson (d.), for their passion, resourcefulness and resolve.

Despite the trend toward virtual libraries, I love the fact that books are living things. They offer an experience that is tangible and tactile. Simultaneously, they are time-limited. They become emblems of the past, as new knowledge supersedes the old. By the time this book is published, many new conversations and research initiatives will have forged ahead. Both challenge and opportunity lie before us in how we name these new initiatives, how we investigate new phenomena and how we understand dance. To continue to live this richness, I proceed with a sense of deep humility and gratitude.

Glenna Batson

Preface

A preface by definition is brief. Ideally, it guides the reader through the aim and scope of a book. Admittedly, this Preface is longer than usual. We ask readers to bear with us. The 'territory' bears fresh tracks, and we've placed signposts along the way to ease navigation.

The theme of this book is embodied cognition in dancemaking.[1] Over the last few decades, the topic has advanced toward a trans-disciplinary discourse. These five main trends are contributing to the current momentum:

1. The accumulated investigations of dance scholars over the twentieth century on the sociocultural and political aspects of the body and embodiment, the self and inter-subjectivity
2. The dialogue between dance and somatic education (Somatics) on movement praxis, profoundly influencing concepts of bodily accessibility and control
3. The accretion of theories on embodiment, bringing consilience to diverse disciplines within the arts, sciences and humanities
4. The rise of dance science as a formal and living tool for dance wellness and injury prevention
5. Advances in digital technologies and behavioral methods of movement analysis, shedding light on cognitive processes within the creation of new movement material[2]

Dance has long subscribed to thinking as embodied. Thinking in dance is shaped by the performative – the intention to communicate art through movement dynamics. Over the twentieth century, dance scholars largely drew from phenomenology, aesthetics and sociocultural studies in reflecting on embodiment in dance. Somatic education (Somatics) deepened these concepts through praxis. While dance gained mightily from this legacy, the value of embodied processes rarely had been framed as *cognitive*.

Over the latter part of the twentieth century as well, embodiment theory took hold within cognitive neuroscience. Today, embodied cognitive neuroscience is a contemporary 'science of intersubjectivity' (Thompson 2001: 1). Cognition results from experience – from dynamic worldly engagement and interaction. The brain needs a world to make thought.

Dancemaking is a *particular* kind of worldly engagement.[3] Its meaning lies in the particularities of transmission – the unique processes by which embodiment is expressed in performance. Lately, dance has captured the interest of scientists and other scholars interested in these processes – more so perhaps than any other sport or movement study. As a living laboratory, dance renders implicit processes explicit and visible. Approximately fifteen years ago, choreographers looked to brain science for creative inspiration as well as to gain another perspective into the processes of dancemaking. '[C]horeographic cognition'[4] has blossomed into an axis of synthetic research in 'artscience' (Edwards 2010). What began as solitary projects has gained global connectivity. Collaborations – both formal and informal – have flourished throughout various parts of the world. A nexus of collaborators is surfacing both within and outside the academy – artists, scientists, digital media experts, dance scholars and teachers. Participants are developing multiple competencies and skills, exploiting new tools and methodologies that benefit the collective in sustainable ways. The exchange is forging a shared language of movement dynamics. New research models are not merely applied, but practice-driven (Borgdorff 2006; Nelson 2013).

This book offers a series of perspectives on this topic from the particular vantage point of Somatics and dance science. The essays are designed to weave together diverse historical and theoretical threads in an evolving conversation on embodied cognition in dancemaking. First, we aim to inform readers on key topics in this emergent exchange in order to deepen discussion across disciplines. What sparked these conversations between dancemakers and the wider body of brain researchers? Why are they important? What avenues are possible for developing a trans-disciplinary approach to research? Second, we revisit the value of somatic education in training embodied cognition in dancemaking. What cognitive studies best support its pedagogical value?

Our book traces the history of embodied cognitive theory in science and points out key events in the evolution of the current dance-science engagement. We briefly review the historical evolution of embodied cognition within cognitive science.[5] Additionally, we categorize current research approaches and projects, bolster the evidence for somatic education within embodied cognitive theory, invite critique, offer practical exercises and garner resources for further research. While informal collaborations between dancers and scientists have flourished, we mainly reference published works and Internet sites specific to embodied cognition in dance.

The study of embodiment is huge. As a relatively new science of human experience and interaction, embodied cognition partakes of the phenomenological and the neurological. This neuro-phenomenological perspective embraces all aspects of autonomous, self-regulatory control within artistic practice and performance. It necessitates a confluence of disciplines – philosophy, cultural studies, human movement science and cognitive neuroscience (human, robotic, artificial and virtual).

Focusing solely on *cognition* leaves us with a wealth of subjects critical to dancemaking: perception, attention, problem-generating and problem-solving, judgment, decision-making and memory…processes integral to the work of the dancing bodymind. Cognitive studies include (but are not limited to) dynamic systems theory and complexity science, human ecology, eco-psychology and ecological dynamics, kinesthesia and kinesthetic empathy, neuroaesthetics, social and affective neuroscience, developmental- and neuropsychology, motor control and motor learning, and a host of other psychophysical and behavioral topics.

Choosing from this vast array, we've extracted three over-arching themes that reflect our vantage point:

1. Embodiment
2. Enaction
3. Attention

Taken together, we revisit these themes in light of theories in embodied cognition and contemporary dancemaking. Further, we've chosen these themes because they call upon the best of our own expertise – the sum of our experience in dance, somatic education and neuroscience. Our aim is to advance the discourse and stimulate new research. To this end, the book supports the work of dance artists, dance scientists, movement teachers, and somatic practitioners as well as the growing subset of neuroscientists engaged in this area of trans-disciplinary research.

To better situate the discussion, we clarify several key terms used throughout the book as follows:

First, the term *dance* in dancemaking: we define dance primarily from the many forms of mid-twentieth-century western contemporary dance. This dance is largely destined for display. This intention shapes cognitive processes uniquely.

Further, while dance (and arguably all movement) is inter-subjective and embodied, western contemporary dance from this period has been informed and enriched by five decades of exchange with Somatics. The dialogue with Somatics has given rise to new dance forms and approaches to pedagogy, blurring boundaries. Somatically informed dance also is subject to global influences that further stretch these boundaries.

Second, we prefer using the terms *body* and *embodiment* instead of *Soma* and *somatic*. Researchers can more readily locate these terms in neuroscience. The word *somatic* has a completely different connotation in medical science, referring primarily to body-based symptoms in medical illness. Further, Thomas Hanna pioneered the term Somatics (from Soma and somatic) in the 1970s. The original context and terminology largely privileged awareness to sensory feedback from the unified inner body and movement experience. By choosing the term *body* we imply the phenomenal multiplicity of possible bodies, as well as the act of making a body. In this sense, body retains its connotations within post-positivist science as environmentally situated, as well as shaped by, sociocultural and technological forces. As such, the dancemaking body is an expression of the inseparable, interrelationship of multiple bodies, minds, contexts and tasks in realizing dance.

On the other hand, we are aware of the limitations in our use of the terms *body* and *embodiment*. By attempting to stay within one historical branch of embodied cognition, we must omit discussion on other important forms of embodiment, such as technological extension. At times, we allude to the value of technology in extending embodiment. Nonetheless, we leave this important offshoot of embodiment theory to other cross-disciplinary experts.[6]

Finally, the term 'neuroscience' in the book's subtitle reflects a particular branch of science – *embodied cognitive* neuroscience. Embodied cognition postulates that thinking arises from – and is shaped by – *experience* – the enacting body within its context. Embodied cognitive neuroscience represents more than three generations of research within cognitive science. The theory of embodied cognition issued largely from the work of biologist and cognitive neuroscientist Francisco Varela, who wrote expansively on this topic across decades (Varela, Thompson and Rosch 1991). While embodied cognitive science is recognized as a distinct science from neuroscience, today it incorporates theories from neuroscience and its many offshoots, such as neuropsychology, social and affective neuroscience.

The book's title derives from the concept that body and mind are unified *by* and *through* movement experience in all its dynamism. We have chosen to use the term 'body *and* mind (in motion)', rather than, perhaps a less dualist *bodymind* or *mind-body*. This choice offers readers the rare opportunity both to parse out key constituents of embodiment and to reintegrate them again within the context of dance.

The subtitle *conversation* implies that what is happening between somatically informed dance and cognitive neuroscience is emergent and not yet a full-fledged discourse. The question still remains as to whether dance and neuroscience are 'two worlds approaching' [each other or] 'two approaches to the same world of movement' (Bläsing, Puttke and Schack 2010: 1). Both fields await a substantive enough body of research, a tested methodology and a blended language to merit the full title of discourse.

The chapters are organized as a series of essays. We introduce each essay with a brief overview and a series of questions that guide the reader toward chapter contents. Topical threads bring forward new perspectives for scholars interested in furthering their professional creative practice. Readers also will find a series of questions to guide further inquiry and experiential explorations complementing the themes in each chapter. These explorations comprise a basic rubric for understanding embodied cognition as having classroom utility for dancemakers. Figures, graphics, tables and photographs provide visual clarity. Resources lead the reader toward more in-depth study.

The Introduction is a personal and historical vignette of how this book came into being. Batson time-travels over the last 35 years of her professional career in a quest to bring dance, somatic education and science under one congenial umbrella.

Chapter 1 offers a brief overview of the history of cognitive science in developing an *embodiment hypothesis* – a theory that opened a compatible meeting ground for dancemakers and neuroscientists.

Chapter 2 introduces key conversations and exchanges in the last fifteen years that have broadened the playing field.

Chapter 3 describes and illustrates a task-based approach to researching embodied cognitive processes in dancemaking.

Chapter 4 revisits the term *embodiment* within dancemaking in light of embodied cognitive theory. The chapter locates the origins of the term *embodied cognition*, alluding to its relevance for dance-science research today.

Chapter 5 revisits the topic of kinesthesis within dancemaking. The chapter posits *enaction theory* as a neuro-phenomenological approach to reframing this topic.

Chapter 6 is the first of four companion chapters on embodied cognitive process. This first chapter is on attention and explores the interrelationship between attention and effort in optimizing physical performance. This chapter sets the stage for advancing a perspective on the effectiveness of somatic education in training attention within dance.

Chapter 7 outlines the elements common to somatic learning environments that are conducive to training embodied attention.

Chapter 8 reviews current theory on the mental practice of motor imagery (in relation to its *sister* practice Ideokinesis) and its relevance to dance. In both practices, visual attention stimulates changes in neuromuscular patterning.

Chapter 9 describes a contrasting somatic approach to training attention we've named 'Somatic Grounding'. This process involves attending to tactile and kinesthetic sensations from movement feedback in promoting postural control and balance.

Chapter 10 offers an experiential narrative on ecological dynamics. Wilson provides insights into *vertical dancing* and how this challenging environment shapes the dancer's attention.

Chapter 11 summarizes the issues facing the engagement between dance and cognitive studies, and poses questions for the road ahead.

The appendices offer the reader a primer on balance as well as reflected questions and self-guided explorations and examples pertinent to each chapter.

To write a book like this means to make choices of what to put in and what to leave out. We write about what most deeply touches our passion: the convergence of dance, Somatics and science. When ideas crystallize between all three, the confluence is nothing less than thrilling. Tackling this emergent discourse in light of our expertise has been humbling. Any one of the disciplines might have been enough but, together, they represent great breadth and depth and an enduring connection to dance movement processes. We realize also, that our perspectives primarily derive from our American- and Eurocentric dance experience. We ask that readers stay poised with open and agile minds in reading these perspectives. Perspectives are not answers, but ways of probing the status quo. In the end, the book is poised along an ongoing trajectory of evolution within dancemaking. To this end, we invite dialogue and debate.

Glenna Batson and Margaret Wilson

References

Bläsing, B., Puttke, M. and Schack, T. (2010), *The Neurocognition of Dance: Mind, Movement and Motor Skills*, New York: Psychology Press.

Borgdorff, H. (2006), 'The Debate on Research in the Arts', http://www.gu.se/digitalAssets/1322/ 1322713_the_debate_on_research_in_the_arts.pdf. Accessed 20 August 2013.

deLahunta, S. (2013), 'Publishing choreographic ideas', in Boxberger, E. and Wittmann, G. (eds.), *pARTnering Documentation: Approaching Dance, Heritage, Culture*. 3rd Dance Education Biennae 2012 Frankfurt am Main. Munchen, DE: Epodium Verlag, pp. 18–25.

Edwards, D. (2010), *Artscience: Creativity in the Post-Google Generation*, Cambridge, MA: Harvard University Press.

Glass, R. and Stevens, C. (2005), 'Choreographic cognition: Investigating the psychological processes involved in creating and responding to contemporary dance', http://ausdance.org .au/articles/details/choreographic-cognition. Accessed 2 April 2014.

Nelson, R. (2013), 'From practitioner to practitioner-researcher', Podcast, Brunel Performance Research Seminar, 13 February 2013. http://www.dance-tech.net/main/search/search?q= robin+nelson+practice+research. Accessed 20 September 2013.

Reynolds, D., Jola, C. and Pollick, F. (2012), 'Editorial introduction & abstracts: Dance and neuroscience – new partnerships', *Dance Research*, 69, pp. 260–69.

Risner, D. (2000), 'Making dance, making sense: Epistemology and choreography', *Research in Dance Education*, 1: 2, pp. 155–172.

Thompson, E. (ed.) (2001), *Between Ourselves: Second-Person Issues in the Study of Consciousness*, Charlottesville, VA: Imprint Academic.

Varela, F.J., Thompson, E. and Rosch, E. (1991), *The Embodied Mind: Cognitive Science and Human Experience*, Cambridge, MA: MIT Press.

Notes

1 The suffix *making* in dancemaking emphasizes the generative capacity and agency within dance choreography – not as thing or product, but as an embodied act of deliberate aesthetic transmission across all phases of the evolution of a dance. Thus, the term implies a range of acts (dancing and choreographing), roles, jobs, competencies and contexts for dance makers. Many universities use the terms 'dance maker' for 'dancer', or 'dance making' for 'dancing' to indicate perhaps a more active participation in creative process. For examples, see Texas Woman's University (http://www.twu.edu/dance/) and the BA program at Coventry University (UK) called Dance Making and Performance (http://www. coventry.ac.uk/course-structure/2013/school-of-art-and-design/undergraduate-degree/ dance-making-and-performance-ba-hons/). See also http://www.danceducationweb .org/performance.html and http://artsalive.ca/en/dan/make/, and Doug Risner's article, 'Making dance, making sense' (Risner 2000). Here, we choose the unhyphenated term 'dancemaking' to suggest not only the unity of the bodymind in the process of making dances, but also the indivisibility of dancer, task and context within the multiplicity of cognitive processes.

2 For a review of trends and examples of emergent dance-science research, see Reynolds, Jola and Pollick 2012 and deLahunta 2013.

3   Embodied cognition in dancemaking is a quintessential example of bodymind unity. Dance gives rise to rich narratives that challenge dualism and even the concept of 'field' or discipline, itself. This is not only true of dance, but also of its sister informant – somatic movement studies. Further, the authors acknowledge 'spiritual' unity in the bodymind integration, but we do not address this topic explicitly.

4   The term 'choreographic cognition' was coined first by psychologist Catherine (Kate) Stevens and dancemaker Shirley McKechnie to describe their collaborative research on the cognitive processes of dancemaking throughout the 1990s (Glass and Stevens 2005).

5   The term 'embodied cognition' was coined by scientist Francisco Varela and his colleagues in 1991 (Varela, Thompson and Rosch, 1991: 147). The roots of the term date back to Varela's work in the late 1960s, when Varela was mentored by biologist Humberto Maturana. See Chapter 4 on embodiment for elaboration.

6   There is neither enough expertise nor space in this book to cover the whole field of embodiment, particularly that corpus which focuses on interactive and extended technologies. Good reviews include: Birringer, J. (2007), 'Performance and science', PAJ 85, pp. 22–35; Kolcio, K. (2005), 'A somatic engagement of technology', *International Journal of Performance Arts and Digital Media*, 1(2), pp. 101–25; Kozel, S. (2007), *Closer: Performance, Technologies, Phenomenology*, Cambridge, MA: The MIT Press; Lycouris, S. (2009), 'Choreographic environments: new technologies and movement-related artistic work', in J. Butterworth and L. Wildschut (eds.), *Contemporary Choreography: A Critical Reader*, London: Routledge, pp. 346–61; de Spain, K. (2011), 'Improvisation and Intimate Technologies', *Choreographic Practices*, 2, pp. 25–42; Schiphorst, T. (2009), 'The varieties of user experience: Bridging embodied methodologies from Somatics and performance to human computer interaction', Ph.D. Thesis, Plymouth, UK: University of Plymouth; and the special issue on Somatics, dance and technology in *Journal of Dance and Somatic Practices*, 2013, 5: 1.

Introduction

In theory, there is no difference between theory and practice…but, in practice, there is.

(Yogi Berra, baseball player, Baseball Hall of Fame, USA)

Time-traveling

The seeds for writing this book were sown more than twenty years ago. Back then, a powerful vision stirred my imagination of an art-science discourse. To realize this vision, I spent my career reconciling differences between disparate knowledge bodies – dance, Somatics, rehabilitation medicine and neuroscience. Today, nearly half a century of dance-science investigation lies behind me. I have lived through a period of enormous social change, witnessing the felling of objective truths and dissolution of unidimensional disciplines. In this Introduction, I wish to highlight key events within dance, Somatics and science that span the 1970s to the present. To this end, I've taken the liberty of embedding my personal experience in these events to ground the book's perspectives within a larger historical context.

In retrospect, I see one concept uniting these disparate knowledge bodies: *self-regulation*.[1] I would not have thought of this term back in the 1970s when I began a serious personal and professional inquiry into dance education. In retrospect, though, issues of self-regulation and control shaped my thirst for learning and my life's journey for the next four decades. Even today, self-regulation may not readily surface as a term of art in dance discussions. Yet, it is as critical to surviving as an artist as it is to thriving as a human being (Skinner 2008; Lobo and Winsler 2006).

Self-regulation is how we control ourselves through flexible and adaptive self-guidance. Self-regulatory theory finds its niche in a number of fields from psychology to cybernetics. While not a biological given, self-regulation arises out of our phenomenal embodiment. Self-regulation calls for a conscious commitment to turn inappropriate and ill-fitting reactions into viable responses. It arises out of learning to discern and reflect on all relationships, both material and transcendent. Vital to sustainable living, self-regulation is how humans endure.

But how do dancers self-regulate? Through what processes do dancers gain skillful *control* over their bodies? In my case, when I was learning to dance, I experienced conflict over how to accomplish the desired movements. As a consequence, my body was riddled with tension. Movement appeared the ultimate paradox: controlled and control-less, consciously aware and oblivious, autonomous and guided, intentional and automatic, reflexive and voluntary, flexible and constrained. While I believed that freedom of movement was my birthright, I had no idea how to arrive at this naturally. How could I exercise constructive control in learning disciplined movement forms without imposing effortful and interfering thoughts? It would take decades before my questions were answered to any degree of self-satisfaction.

An early vignette

I learned a great deal about self-regulation through my first formal physical training: modern dance. The cultural milieu of modern dance in the 1950s was grounded in a disciplined aesthetic that inspired in me a deep love of expressive movement. I was born in 1948, and grew up in a dancing family. My mother danced with Ruth St. Denis and Hanya Holm.[2] This rich legacy etched its way into my being and undoubtedly altered my DNA. I recall the way my mother embodied Miss Ruth – her bearing, her reverent vocabulary and gestures, the way dance helped her escape from the banality of human existence, her interest in theosophy and her exotic costumes and music. For years, I lived with the daily drumbeat of Hanya's percussive pulse in my mother's studio. While more traditional mothers of that time stayed anchored to their aprons in the kitchen, my mother was dancing the Balinese Legong at the local US Army Officers' Club. The costume room in the basement of our house was a sacred temple of mystery and magic. Here, even into my teenage years, I'd hide from the conformity of my peers with their loafers and pleated skirts, prancing around in headdresses, veils and heels. While I enjoyed swingin' to the rock 'n' roll music of my generation, my most revered hours were spent in rapt improvisation to dissonant 78-rpm anthologies from the Far East.

Although my mother discouraged me from becoming a dancer, I nevertheless craved this life. I pursued it against all odds. My formal studies included many forms of dance: classical ballet, modern dance techniques from Graham to Hawkins, jazz, tap, multiple ethnic (folk) forms and even baton-twirling. Despite the richness of offerings, I was dissatisfied with the *do as I do* form of transmission in teaching and my own stumbling blocks in learning. Teachers relied largely on mimicking and repetition strategies. Mirrors were everywhere, and I did not like what I saw. I was not particularly gifted, either physically or cosmetically. My awkwardness was combined with an abnormal dose of self-consciousness and angst about not looking the part or doing the *right* thing.

While I loved my teachers for their earnestness and dedication, their classes provided few answers to my longing for movement freedom. I believed such freedom must be only a whisper away, yet I was struck by its elusiveness. Often, a teacher's stylistic movement choices seemed irrelevant and illogical. Every move seemed like the wrong fit for my body. I would tacitly ask myself, 'Why are we doing this?' I struggled mightily to do as instructed, but often ended tied up in an anatomical straightjacket by my habitual tensions and mental armoring. Unable to find a physical inroad into movement coordination naturally, I would try to use an analytical approach to solve my movement problems, not realizing that such mental effort kept me farther away from movement freedom than ever. I remained a troubled student for decades.

In retrospect, I realize that I was seeking a unified perspective that would satisfy my aesthetic and intellectual curiosity while affording me access to my own bodily ease. Of all my dance teachers, I was particularly drawn to Erick Hawkins, whose crystalline mind crafted the logic of his technique without sacrificing his art. Hawkins saw art and science as 'complementary polarities of direction…analogous to the two ways of knowing the world – the one, through immediate apprehension; the other, through the theoretical, as in science. It takes both to complete our knowledge of the world. Science itself uses both, as does art' (Hawkins 1992: 26). I studied with Erick and his teachers in the late 1970s and early 1980s. It became clear during this period, though, that I was not destined for a career in dance performance but rather for another – yet unknown – role within dance.

Enter Somatics: the 1970s

The 1960s and 1970s gave rise to a number of sociocultural shifts that offered me a personal – and ultimately, a professional – outlet to my frustrations. Many counterculture – and protest movements marked this period – the Vietnam anti-war movement, the Civil Rights movement and women's liberation, to name a few. Postmodern dance and the Somatics movement also proliferated during this period.

Somatic education really needs no introduction to dancers. The praxis dialogue between western dance and Somatics finds its origins in the early part of the twentieth century. Here is an enormous praxis archive on the dynamics of self-regulation. The ethos of both these practices was the dismembering of dualism between body and mind, and the freedom of bodily expression. Both dance and Somatics reacted against puritanical and reductionist views of the body. Both celebrated bodily sensuality and sensitivity. Both promised to unleash movement potential – its generative power, its efficiency and its self-organizing properties – although initially through very different means.

What might not be apparent to dancers is that Somatics pioneer Thomas Hanna (1928–90) argued for Somatics as a science of self-regulation as early as 1973. Within the spectrum of the humanistic psychology movement, Hanna advocated for the science of 'Somatology' (Hanna 1973). This science, Hanna believed, would help undo centuries of Cartesian dualism and empower personal, first-person experience and self-regulation,[3] both in the scientific arena and in public education. Hanna was prescient in regarding first-person experience as the valid source of self-regulation. He distinguished between moral philosophy and natural philosophy. While Hanna deemed moral philosophy outside the bounds of science, he saw natural philosophy as capable of evolving into a science, whose goal was not toward an abstraction of truth and beauty. Rather, this new 'science' was grounded in the conscious awareness of one's own experience. It promised freedom and empowerment.

Somatics works on a different scale than dance. Here, movers sensitize to subtle messages arising from micro-dynamics of movement. Attending consciously to these micro-movements and micro-processes fosters bodymind integration. In this milieu, non-conscious, automatic processes of self-regulation can surface more readily in an atmosphere free of the usual trappings of habitual patterns of effort. Within Somatics, there is less need to achieve movement goals or anticipate outcomes. The methods replace willful doing with listening and attuning to process. Within dance, this kind of attention shifts consciousness away from the *what* of learning (the steps or vocabulary) to the *how* (bodymind processes).[4]

For me, Somatics provided powerful insights into autonomous self-regulation. These approaches offered a safe, intuitive, pleasurable means of uncovering the mysteries of *control*. I spent the next few decades deeply steeped in Somatics. I owe an enormous debt to my first teacher in somatic learning: Irene Dowd. I studied with Irene intensively between 1977 and 1982. I had gone to her first to get help with a poorly rehabilitated injury. Although the initial trauma of the injury was over, I still was nearly incapacitated from pain and dysfunction despite several years of medical treatment. At the time, Irene was emerging from her position of protégé to Dr. Lulu Sweigard (Ideokinesis) at Julliard Conservatory, and was advancing her own work in 'kinesthetic anatomy'.[5] Kinesthetic anatomy was a vital portal of entry into understanding my own body – not only my body's parts and functions, but also through embodied movement experience. Creatively linking didactic with experiential learning unleashed my body's transformative potential, fusing structure and function in one aesthetic. Irene inspired in me a love for science as a co-partner with art in understanding movement.

Learning Ideokinesis was my first formal attempt at understanding the interrelationship of effort and coordination. Herein was a body of knowledge whose principles concurred with those emerging in science. As well, Ideokinesis provided a practical and pragmatic route to understanding the art of self-regulation. Ideokinesis further afforded me a catalyst for embodied learning, self-development and creativity. From my collaborations with Irene, I evolved into a somatic educator. Far from a cookie-cutter trade, her instruction was an apprenticeship of head, hand and heart. I would become a transmitter of embodied knowledge, helping others become more of themselves through embodied movement learning.

From the 1970s to the end of the millennium, dance and Somatics found a common ethos through directed kinesthetic awareness of movement dynamics. Initially, however, the primary intentions differed between the two. Dance arguably aimed toward aesthetic expression and Somatics toward health and wellbeing (Volkers 2007). Perhaps because of these different intentions, the pedagogy diverged for quite some time. Placing sensory awareness in the foreground was radical in more traditional western contemporary dance pedagogy. The significance of the first-person inner narrative as both content and method was an affront to the reigning pedagogy.[6] Dance training drew largely from conditioning methods – copying the teacher, memorizing steps, and repeating and reinforcing steps and phrases, often in front of mirrors. While these methods still have validity today, at that time, a culture of rigor prevailed in which becoming a true artist was linked to the degree of physical and emotional suffering endured.[7]

With the continuing praxis dialogue between dance and Somatics, and increasing diversification within both disciplines, both means and ends became more fused over time. Privileging the sensory in first-person movement experience gave rise to an empowering unity of mind and body. Rather than viewing the body as instrument or vehicle, Somatics viewed the body as contextual and fluid. A more optimal relationship between body and mind could more likely thrive in an environment in which the (s)pace of learning allowed for autonomous movement exploration – control lay in the process (the means), while suspending the movement outcome (the goal).

Enter dance science: the 1980s

From the 1970s onward, I pursued various forms of somatic education as a means of personal and professional development. This pursuit was profoundly rewarding to all dimensions of my life, including my dancing. Professionally, however, I was stymied by the uni-disciplinary approach to career development that was characteristic of that time: dance *or* science, dance *or* Somatics, or, from its most oppositional vantage point, dance *vs.* science and dance science *vs.* Somatics. I longed for a different language – corporeal and incorporating. *Trans*-disciplinarity was a distant dream that was going to require time – decades, in fact – of scholarly evolution.

In 1977, I entered a Masters degree program in dance education at Columbia University Teachers College in New York. By 1978, I was working as a *movement therapist* for Dr. Richard Bachrach, DO who specialized in working with performing artists. Richard was a maverick in his interest in performing arts medicine. He believed enough in my ability to hire me as a movement coach with only a Masters in dance education (*sans* a professional medical license). I worked with Richard for two years as a specialist in movement (re-)education. We established a dance medicine clinic, inviting dancers in for weekly educational sessions on anatomy and injury prevention.

This period saw the formal establishment of *dance science* with the formation of the International Association of Dance Medicine & Science (IADMS) (www.iadms.org). Richard and I would present together on the iliopsoas and back pain at the first IADMS conference in 1984 in New York City. The formation of the IADMS was vital for the advancement of science within dance. For the first time, a coalition of physicians (mainly orthopedists and osteopaths), physical therapists and dance educators found common themes around injury prevention and safe and effective dance training. In the beginning, however, the field had its own particular ethos (Green 2001; Green 2007). In the effort to establish a scientific foundation for dance teaching and performance, dance scientists sought to find a rationale for safe and effective dance training within scientific theory. These sciences initially included sports and exercise science, biomechanics and kinesiology, psychology, nutrition, anatomy, motor learning, motor control and motor development, orthopedics, rehabilitation medicine and other related fields within science and medicine.

Despite the sizeable goodwill early on, the dialogue between dance science and Somatics admittedly was difficult (Batson, Wilson and Quin 2012). Positivist models of scientific research also created tensions, appearing awkward, limited or downright incompatible in capturing the scope of human movement. Dance readily posed a significant challenge to those framing artistic movement performance as science.[8] Scientific rhetoric seemed inflexible and reductionist; quantifiable models failed to capture implicit processes and spatiotemporal dynamics. A tacit prejudice that science somehow ruins art (and/or that dancers do not have the capacity for science), stymied interdisciplinary communication (Krasnow 2005). Likewise, somatic vocabulary seemed irreducibly subjective. It seemed impossible to generalize from personal narratives. Such subjectivity was fraught with jargon, ultimately ungeneralizable and therefore, unscientific. Somatics introduced words like *mind-body* and *living consciousness* – words far removed from the terminology used by positivist science research and allopathic medicine. Critics claimed that somatic approaches lacked evidence of their effectiveness. The actual dearth of scientific studies left Somatics marginalized within the field, even at the level of discussion.

Wherever dance was happening, however, the atmosphere was stunningly open to somatic investigation. The exploratory atmosphere was electric, illuminating new pathways for growth, teaching and learning. I left New York in 1980 to teach in the dance department at the University of Maryland, a context in which I was ill suited. I was struggling with a poorly rehabilitated injury, and faced too many limitations to evolve into the teacher or performer I envisioned. I was still passionate, however, about linking dance with Somatics and science, so I sought another route. I went on to pursue a degree in physical therapy in 1983. This would begin another long period of striving for integration between disparate bodies of knowledge.

Embodiment confluence: the 1990s

The late 1980s through the 1990s was a period of enormous paradigm shift that brought art and science into closer confluence. Embodiment became the '*grande idée*' over the next decade; the fostering nexus of focused research that inspired a renaissance within the academy (after Bresler 2004: 4). This was an exciting period of confluence between the arts, humanities, science and technology. Sociocultural, artistic and scientific ramifications of body and embodiment created a move toward consilience within many fields.[9]

Interdisciplinarity broke down rigid barriers within the academy and opened up multiple vantage points to new ways of thinking. Dance scholarship thrived during this period through a broad spectrum of approaches to embodiment – dance phenomenology, sociocultural and sociopolitical perspectives, performance studies, somatic studies and dance science. Dance research also became infused with post-positivist theory and reflexive methodologies. By the late 1990s, Somatics had enriched embodiment scholarship through a host of pragmatic practices. These influences shifted the study of dance toward embodied process and enabled researchers to begin to measure what was heretofore immeasurable.[10]

By the end of the 1990s, many elements of somatic education were filtered into the dance classroom worldwide. New dance forms proliferated globally (most notably, Contact Improvisation). Many dancers today have become somatic practitioners, deepening their work as artists and teachers. Numerous academic (and non-academic) programs now offer advanced degrees and certificates qualifying dancers in somatic studies. After many decades of exploring various avenues of exchange, the conversation between dance and Somatics has become richly interwoven and their principles and practices merged. The term somatically informed dance praxis (and vice versa, dance informed Somatics) more readily reveals their confluence. At the same time, critique continues to enliven the discussion (Green 2007).

In 1986, I spent a summer with Bonnie Bainbridge-Cohen at the first certification course in Body-Mind Centering. In 1987, I attended Naropa Institute where I first had classes with Nancy Stark Smith. Nancy's approach to the improvisational physics of Contact Improvisation was electrifying. That summer I also met biologist and cognitive neuroscientist Francisco Varela. I was dazzled by Varela's brilliant exposition of *autopoiesis* – his theory of the autonomous and enacting nature of biological intelligence. These teachers were saying similar things – just with very different vocabularies.

That same summer, Martha Myers began organizing intensives that brought together dance scientists and somatic practitioners to the ADF. I participated as a workshop leader in a number of summer offerings. This was to be the start of a quarter of a century of association with the festival. I taught for the Hollins/ADF M.F.A. program from its inception in 2006 until 2013, gradually morphing course content of *Contemporary Body Practices* from a survey of Somatics in 2006, to an exploration of neuroscientific theory around embodied cognition in dancemaking.

Toward embodiment science

As I write this book, I see that my own approaches to teaching reflect the wider scope of change in the sociocultural landscape. This last quarter century has witnessed enormous shifts in every sector of societal interchange. Postmodern trends within dance performance, Somatics and science have given way to the shifting tides of *transmodernism*.[11] Inter-disciplinary perspectives on the self, embodiment, complexity and control have evolved toward trans-disciplinarity. More than ever, a confluence of theoreticians and pragmatic movers are partnering with one another to break down barriers, hierarchies and binding structures, and opening to new influences. We find ourselves bridging across formerly incompatible distances in new and exciting ways (Shaughnessy 2013). Discussions on cognitive process are themselves a process of co-creation in a quest for a deeper understanding of the reciprocity of body and mind in motion. Conceptual fluidity shifts the focus from the hegemony of brain science or the science of mind to symbiotic investigations within a more level playing field of 'cognitive studies.' (McConachie and Hart 2006: ix). The meshing of theory and practice provides fresh insights into how brain, mind and the performative body inter-relate. As this meshed space enlarges to embrace the un-fragmented gestalt of movement experience, terminological boundaries morph towards increased clarity. The perspectives in this book address some of the challenges in this evolution. Read on.

References

Bagioli, M. (1995), 'Tacit knowledge, courtliness, and the scientist's body', in S.L. Foster (ed.), Bloomington, IN: Indiana University Press, pp. 69–81.

Batson, G. (1990), 'Dancing fully, safely and expressively: The role of Somatics in dance education', *Journal of Physical Education, Recreation and Dance*, 61: 9, pp. 28–31.

Batson, G. and Schwartz, R.E. (2007), 'Revisiting the value of somatic education in dance training through an inquiry into practice schedules', *Journal of Dance Education*, 7: 2, pp. 47–56.

Batson, G. Wilson, M.A. and Quin, E. (2012), 'Integrating somatics and science', *Journal of Dance and Somatic Practices*, 3: 1–2, pp. 183–93.

Beavers, W. (2008), 'Locating technique', in M. Bales and R. Nettl-Fiol (eds.), *The Body Eclectic: Evolving Practices in Dance Training*, Urbana, IL: University of Illinois Press, pp. 126–33.

Berger, A. (2011), *Self-Regulation: Brain, Cognition and Development*, Washington, DC: Imprint.

Berrol, C.F. (2004), 'How to mix quantitative and qualitative and methods in a dance/movement therapy research project', in R.F. Cruz and C.F. Berrol (eds.), *Dance Movement Therapists in Action: A Working Guide to Research Options*, Springfield, IL: Charles C. Thomas, Publisher, pp. 233–52.

Bresler, L. (ed.) (2004), *Knowing Bodies, Moving Minds: Towards Embodied Teaching and Learning*, London: Kluwer Academic Publishers.

Cole, M. (2008), *Marxism and Educational Theory: Origins and Issues*. London: Routledge.

Daston, L. and Galison, P. (2007), *Objectivity*, Cambridge, MA: MIT Press.

Dussel, E. (1995), *The Invention of the Americas: Eclipse of 'the Other' and the Myth of* Modernity. M.D. Barber (trans.) http://biblioteca.clacso.edu.ar/ar/libros/dussel/1492in/1492in.html. Accessed 23 March 2014.

Farrugia, K. (2012), *Transmodern Dance Practices: Angelin Preljocaj, Auro Bigozetti and Revisions of Les Noces*. Ph.D. thesis, London Metropolitan University, London: UK.

Fortin, S. (2005), 'Measurable? Immeasurable? What are we looking for?', *Proceedings of the Laban Research Conference Day*, London: Trinity Laban Conservatoire of Music and Dance, pp. 3–8.

Green, J. (2001), 'Socially constructed bodies in American dance classrooms', *Research in Dance Education*, 2: 2, pp. 155–73.

Green, J. (2002), 'Somatics: A growing and changing field', *Journal of Dance Education*, 2: 4, pp. 113–17.

Green, J. (2007), 'Student bodies: Dance pedagogy and the soma', *Springer International Handbook of Research in Arts Education*, 16, pp. 1119–35.

Green, J. and Stinson, S. (1999), 'Positivist research in dance', in S. Fraleigh and P. Hanstein (eds.), *The Art of Research: Systematic Inquiry*, Pittsburgh: University of Pittsburgh Press, pp. 91–102.

Hanna, T. (1973), 'The project of Somatology', *Journal of Humanistic Psychology*, 13: 3, pp. 3–13.

Hanna, T. (1990/1991), 'Clinical somatic education: A new discipline in the field of health care', *Somatics: Magazine-Journal of the Bodily Arts and Sciences*, 8: 1. http://somatics.org/library/clinicalsomatics. Accessed 11 February 2013.

Hawkins, E. (1992), *The Body Is a Clear Place: And Other Statements on Dance*, Princeton, NJ: Princeton Book Company.

Krasnow, D. (2005), 'Sustaining the dance artist: barriers to communication between educators, artists and researchers', in K. Vincs (ed.), *Dance Rebooted: Initializing the Grid*, Conference Proceedings, Ausdance National, December 2004. http://ausdance.org.au/articles/details/sustaining-the-dance-artist. Accessed 28 April 2012.

Lakes, R. (2005), 'The messages behind the methods: The authoritarian pedagogical legacy in Western concert dance technique training and rehearsals', *Arts Education Policy Review*, 106: 5, pp. 3–10.

Lobo, Y.B. and Winsler, A. (2006), 'The effects of a creative dance and movement program on the social competence of head start preschoolers, social development', *Social Development*, 3, pp. 501–19.

McConachie, B. and Hart F. Elizabeth (eds.) (2006), *Performance and Cognition: Theatre Studies and the Cognitive Turn*. New York, NY: Routledge.

Robey, J. (2011), 'Dance paradigms (Part 8: transmodern dance). Blog entry, Friday, November 18, 2011. http://themindfuldancer.blogspot.co.uk/2011/11/dance-paradigms-part-8-transmodern.html. Accessed 23 March 2014.

Rodriguez Madga, R. M. (1989), *La Sonrisa de Satumo: Hacia una Teoria Transmoderna*. Barcelona, Spain: Anthropos.

Shaughnessy, N. (ed.) (2013), *Affective Performance and Cognitive Science: Body, Brain and Being*. New York, NY: Bloomsbury.

Skinner, J. (2008), 'Women dancing back—and forth: Resistance and self-regulation in Belfast Salsa', *Dance Research Journal*, 40: 1, pp. 65–77.

Slingerland, E. and Collard, M. (2011), *Creating Consilience: Integrating the Sciences and the Humanities*, New York, NY: Oxford University Press.

Stinson, S.W. (1995), 'Body of knowledge', *Educational Theory*, 45: 1, pp. 43–54.

Snow, C.P. (1959), *The Two Cultures*, London: Cambridge University Press.

Szaniawski, J. (2004), 'Transmodernism or the resurgence of modernism in contemporary cinema and popular culture', *Belgian Journal of English Language and Literatures*, 2, pp. 167–183.

Volkers, H. (2007), 'Preface', in S. Gehm, P. Husemann and K. von Wilcke (eds.), *Knowledge in Motion: Perspectives of Artistic and Scientific Research in Dance*, New Brunswick, NJ: Transaction Publishers, pp. 3–10.

Wilson, E.O. (1992), *Consilience: The Unity of Knowledge*, New York, NY: Knopf.

Zimmerman, B.J. and Schunk, B.H. (2011), *Handbook of Self-Regulation of Learning and Performance*, New York, NY: Routledge.

Notes

1 For a review of self-regulation, see Zimmerman and Schunk 2011, or Berger 2011.

2 My mother's professional name was Linda Verrill. I have placed her archives, including original correspondence with Ruth St. Denis in the Royal Netherlands Institute for Southeast Asian and Caribbean Studies in the Netherlands: http://www.kitlv.nl/. The Institute graciously accepted the donation.

3   Thomas Hanna's grasp of bodily (somatic) experience as fully integrated with thought is evident in his statement: 'Thought is movement, speech is movement, and it is a movement in concert with all other moving patterns of the "body". If we realistically declare what a "body" is, it is the entire unified system of movements that is ourselves in all our conscious and unconscious functions' (Hanna 1990/1991).

4   These words *what* and *how* are my own, appearing in my article Batson 1990, but I have also found them in Stinson 1995.

5   Irene Dowd first started using this term in the 1970s. I assume it is her own invention.

6   Researcher Dr. Jill Green describes this introduction of Somatics into dance pedagogy as a 'potential minefield' (Green 2002: 114). The novelty of honing sensory acuity in learning movement remains a radical notion to this day in some dance milieus.

7   For elaboration, see Batson and Schwartz 2007; Beavers 2008; and Lakes 2005.

8   The history of the dichotomy of knowledge between art and science is captured best, perhaps, by C.P. Snow (1959). In the 1960s, science was perceived as the only objective reality, while art served to interpret reality. The history of positivist science operated through an ontological presumption of objectivity that aspired to 'a kind of knowledge that bears no trace of the knower...' (Daston and Galison 2010: 17). Objectivity was created to suppress and negate subjectivity. Scientific truth allegedly was 'objective, reducible, and value free' (Green and Stinson 1999: 91). Positivist methodology found utility in hypothesis testing and quantifiable data, demanding a formal distancing from the very subject of engagement. Thus, doing science created its own cultural posturing, a 'stance' likened to that of a seventeenth-century courtier (Bagioli 2009: 74).

9   The term and concept of consilience was developed by E.O. Wilson (1992) and later elaborated by Slingerland and Collard (2011).

10 See Fortin 2005; Green and Stinson 1999; and Berrol 2004, for reviews on merging qualitative and quantitative approaches in dance-Somatics studies.

11 The term 'transmodern' has been attributed first to Spanish philosopher Rosa Maria Rodriguez Magda (1989) in the literature arena. Since then, sociocultural articulations include those by Argentinian philosopher and leftist political theorist Enrique Dussell (1995), film researcher Jeremi Szaniawski (2004), educational theorist Mike Cole (2008), and has been described artistically by Professor James Mahoney of the University of Maryland, Baltimore County as exhibiting three qualities: the liminal, the littoral, and the singularity. For perspectives on aligning transmodernism with dance, see Robey blogspot (2011) and Farrugia (2012).

Chapter 1

From Conversation to Discourse

...the aesthetic has long located art within a science of sensuous knowing. What neurosciences and cognitive science are now adding to the equation is this exciting possibility of getting closer to the underlying conditions fueling that ancient relationship....

(Barbara Stafford 2011: 1)

Overview

At the turn of the twenty-first century, dancers found themselves in a new and compelling conversation around the topic of cognitive processes within dancemaking. The now-global dialogue on embodied cognition has opened a space for artistic and scientific exchange. Synthetic theories and emergent technologies have charted new methodologies for researching embodied processes. The results have been tangible, spawning new movement creation, bolstering interdisciplinary studies and benefiting sociocultural, scientific and medical sectors. This chapter highlights early formal initiatives in this exchange.

Focusing in...

- What topics are dancers currently researching within embodied cognition?
- What exchanges are happening globally in research, choreography and pedagogy?
- What forms are these exchanges taking – artistic, scientific, social/humanitarian, synthetic and beyond?
- What benefits have been realized in different sociocultural and technological sectors?
- What potential obstacles to future development merit our attention?

Experiential prelude

From where do you draw choreographic inspiration outside of dance praxis? How do you work with other fields of study, social networks and digital or other technologies to enhance your growth and development, personally and professionally? Where do you locate your work within history and historicity, from conservation (archiving) at one end to preservation (sustainability) at the other?

Create a 'mind map' – a graphic drawing of your *tree of knowledge*.[1] Are you surprised by the results? Make a list of words that embrace embodied cognition in dancemaking. Now consider these questions: Where are you positioned within this conversation? What challenges do you see within the conversation and exchange? In what ways is dance influencing perspectives on embodiment in science or other disciplines?

Open-sourced dance

'May you live in interesting times' is a colloquial Chinese proverb containing within it the paradox of opportunity and curse. These times are interesting, indeed. Today, globalization and technology are driving a culture of continuous innovation. The message (overt or covert) is a call to constantly change. Within western post-modern dance, this spirit of innovation is a potent modus operandi. The processes of dancemaking have been likened to an irrepressible 'evolutionary urge' (Mason 2009: 27), struggling to thrive through complex processes of selection and variation. One major difference exists, however: Compared to the actual process of Darwinian evolution, the timeline is sped up exponentially.

As various trends continue to shape the evolution of dance, the threat of ossification and extinction loom. Tension exists between preserving the past and future survival (Lansdale 2005). Over the last century, dance has made an enormous impact on social capital and community cohesion. Meta-analyses have shattered the perception of dance as an esoteric, elite discipline devoted solely to art making (Guetzkow 2002; Mitchell, Innoue and Blumenthal 2002; Reid 2011; Burns 2007).

Paradoxically, the impact of continuous innovation offers the promise of sustainability in dance. Simultaneously, it demands that dancers lead 'hybrid lives', (Risner 2012: 185). One emblem of survival has been the thrust towards open-sourced knowledge and interdisciplinarity. Relational and cooperative in its ethos (Warburton 2011), dance largely has challenged single discipline hegemony (Melrose 2009). Throughout the last half of the twentieth century particularly, dancers sourced[2] from everywhere for inspiration and artistic development (Borgdorff 2009). Collaborations have ramified into a system with many interacting parts offering multiple possibilities for connection (Stafford 2011). Dancers engaged in cross-disciplinary, multi-disciplinary, trans-disciplinary, post-disciplinary and even anti-disciplinary collaborations (Liu 2010; Burt 2009). These were remarkable for their heterogeneity, diversity, originality (Borgdorff 2009: 3, 13) and debatable success (Liu 2010). Interdisciplinarity within dance implies that projects have enough body and momentum to survive a contextual flash-in-the-pan.[3] After all, sourcing in dance is not only a matter of acquiring knowledge, but also *embodying* knowledge through dynamical movement processes.

The exchange around cognitive processes in dancemaking is of particular interest. In the last two decades, dance has captured the imagination of many scientists interested in embodiment and cognition, exceeding that of other movement studies (gymnastics, sports or martial arts, for example). Interest in embodied cognition has stretched across a wider spectrum of domains, such as cognitive and affective neuroscience, phenomenology, neuropsychology, human movement science and digital technology. Discourses on embodiment have proliferated and cross-pollenated. Dancemakers now can source from a growing number of sub-disciplines and knowledge bases heretofore unrecognized and inaccessible (Figure 1.1).

Science and its supporting technologies offer dance a unique lens through which to examine dancemaking; dance likewise offers science a dynamic laboratory for investigation. Novel research threads and artistic collaborations have emerged (Bläsing, Puttke and Schack, 2010; Reynolds, Jola and Pollick 2012; Gehm, Husemann, and von Wilcke 2007). Exchanges are co-creating new methodologies, new platforms for exchange and new spaces for discussion and design. The engagement generates new questions in building and sharing competencies (Lapuente 2012; Borgdorff 2009). Whether formal or informal, this engagement has engendered new ideas that bridge across creative processes and research outcomes (Barnard and deLahunta 2011). Two decades of exchange have sown the seeds of new research that is both applied (praxis-based) and praxis-*driven* (Borgdorff 2006; Bläsing et al. 2012; deLahunta, Clarke and Barnard 2012).

The engagement offers mutual inspiration, affirmation and perhaps, confirmation to an understanding of embodied cognitive processes within dance. At the same time, as a new discourse emerges, it faces the challenge of creating a space for standing on its own without

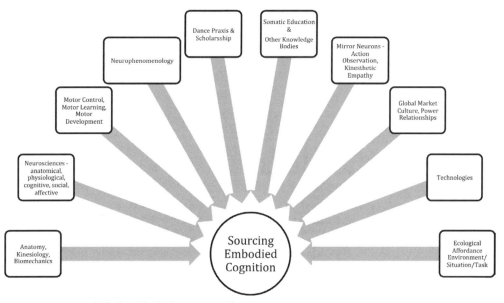

Figure 1.1: Sourcing links for embodied cognitive studies.

17

being dominated by the constraints (language among them) of other fields of knowledge.[4,5] Such exchanges, therefore, call for an ongoing commitment to conceptual flexibility as they strive for rigor within and across their own domains. These collaborations strongly influence scientific as well as artistic values (Birringer and Fenger 2005, deLahunta, Barnard and McGregor 2009; McCarthy et al. 2006).

Dancemaking demands a deep immersion into systems complexity as researchers strive to capture and describe its dynamic processes. Thinking-while-dancing expands our understanding of the human capacity for creativity in communication and design.[6] Via its immediacy of communication, dance provides a powerful, continuously evolving vocabulary for describing complex concepts within its own artistic outpourings, as well as for modeling those in science (Kolcio and Hingorani 2011).

The current conversation raises many evocative questions for all engaged (de Lahunta, Clarke and Barnard 2012) and provokes re-examination and clarification of many concepts (Figure 1.2). Just what cognitive processes in dancemaking are under scrutiny? How successfully have researchers been able to capture these dynamic processes? How might knowledge of these processes inform dance pedagogy, guide learning and enhance performance? How then might a growing understanding of these processes also continue to benefit other sociocultural, scientific and medical realms of inquiry?

We pause in the flow of the current conversation to identify pioneering collaborations contributing to the current momentum in embodied cognition in dancemaking. This chapter recounts pivotal historical events that surfaced at the end of the twentieth century. In addition to listing events, we call attention to the current openings and the barriers to future engagement. The following summary recounts key players and events that have given momentum to the current conversation.

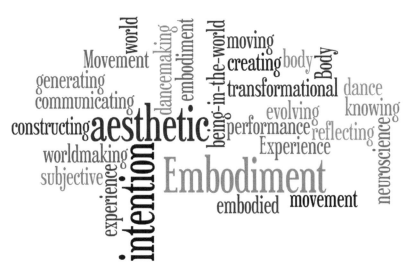

Figure 1.2: *Word Cloud*: Multidisciplinary engagement calls for clarification of shared terms.

Initial visibility

Throughout the latter half of the twentieth century dance scholars stocked their intellectual coffers with scholarship impressive for its breadth of coverage on the topic of embodiment – phenomenological, sociocultural and aesthetic (Sheets-Johnstone, 1981; 1992; 2011; Fraleigh 1991, Lepecki 2004; Cooper-Albright 1997; Kozel, 2007; van Manen 2007; Rouhiainen 2007; Legrand and Ravn 2009 – to name a few!) As phenomenology filtered into brain science (Miller 2003; Paterson 2012), the scientific climate warmed to the idea of embodiment and the moving body's role in thinking.

In the 1990s, Australian cognitive psychologist Catherine Stevens and dancemaker Shirley McKechnie spearheaded a formal investigation into the topic of cognition in dancemaking by coining the term 'choreographic cognition' (Stevens et al. 2003). Over a nine-month period, these dancers recorded their choreographic process. They averaged fifteen hours a week, working with a choreographer in shaping all phases of raw material from inspiration to production of a final 40-minute piece of choreography, *Red Rain* (Stevens et al. 2003). Supported by a grant from the Australian Research Council, the project was a collaboration between the Victorian College of the Arts, the University of Melbourne, Australian Dance Council (Ausdance), the Choreographic Centre, Canberra, and the MARCS Auditory Laboratories and the University of Western Sydney. The collaborators strove to format their creative work as *research*, carefully investigating the literature for methodological precedents on creativity, documenting the process and working with experimental psychologists on developing measurable outcomes. The cohort published extensive results of nearly a decade of dance-science engagement. This body of work was the first comprehensive attempt at articulating the relationship between cognitive and choreographic process (Grove, Stevens and McKechnie 2005; Stevens and McKechnie 2005).

The late 1990s also witnessed a fruitful exchange between dancemakers and scientists in Europe and Australia. Researchers began to tackle complex issues around cognitive processes embedded in the creation of a gestural art form. Formal and informal projects surfaced within the academy and within the professional dance world. Leading the initiatives were key choreographers from Europe and Australia, including William Forsythe (Ballett Frankfurt), Wayne McGregor | Random Dance U.K., and Shirley McKechnie and Catherine Stevens, University of Melbourne. These collaborators not only produced artistic projects in their home base, but also extended their work to distant scientific and artistic centers. In the United Kingdom, Wayne McGregor | Random Dance and dance-science researcher Scott deLahunta collaborated with a group of scientists, philsophers and other thinkers and technicians on a project entitled 'Choreography and Cognition', a project which subsequently included cognitive scientist, David Kirsh, California, US (Kirsh et al. 2009). In Germany, William Forsythe and The Forsythe Company created *Synchronous Objects*, a choreographic project based at The Ohio State University, US.[7]

In the United States of America, interdisciplinary projects in dance and neuroscience began modestly on college campuses. The first published collaboration took place in 2002, at Allegheny College (Pennsylvania). Here, choreographer Bill Evans collaborated with neuroscientists and psychologists at a summer institute called *Neuroscience of Dance and Movement*. Hosted by the campus Neuroscience and Humanities institute, the course featured guest dance artist Evans (teaching Labananalysis) in dialogue with dance director Jan Hyatt, neuropsychology professor Alexander Dale, and psychology professor Jeff Hollerman. The scaffold of inquiry was designed to offer college students without dance backgrounds a chance to capture 'the "whole" of human [movement] experience.' Different knowledge bases were viewed not as 'contradictory but rather…as useful polarities on a continuum…' (Dale, Hyatt and Hollerman 2007: 100).

During this initial decade of cross-disciplinary dialogue, international dance and science symposia began to proliferate. These formal symposia brought together dancers, scientists and other humanities scholars. In the United Kingdom, the Dana Foundation sponsored 'Dance and the Brain,' hosted by Ballett Frankfurt in 2004, and included guest neuroscientists, Marc Jeannerod and Julie Grèzes. In 2006, the Federal Cultural Foundation of Germany organized *Dance Congress Germany*, the first dance congress to be held in over 50 years, looking at the knowledge base of dance – including neuroscience – with the subsequent publishing of *Knowledge in Motion: Perspectives of Artistic and Scientific Research in Dance*. In 2009, the Wellcome Trust (U.K.) hosted a *Research Workshop on Dance and Cognitive Neurosciences*. In Germany, at the University of Bielefeld organized a conference hosted by Tanzplan Essen 2010 on *Intelligence and Action – Dance in the Focus of Cognitive Science* with the subsequent publication of *Tanz im Kopf* (Birringer and Fenger 2005). Investigating how movement and thought co-shape the dance aesthetic brought together many disciplines within brain- and human movement science (Bläsing et al., 2012). With the dawn of the new millennium, researchers were exploring several topics on cognition and dancemaking.[8] Embodied cognition in dancemaking began to appear as a topic of interest in dance medicine conferences and other hybrid symposia on cognition in the arts, sciences and humanities.[9]

Bi-directional[10] research

One shared objective in the current dialogue is 'to seek connections between choreographic processes and the study of movement and the brain/mind that are scientifically and artistically interesting' (deLahunta, Barnard and McGregor 2009). Science needs the perspective of dancers, those whose cognitive problem solving arises out of the movement moment. Dance artists need the perspective of science to reflect rigorously on their processes. Collaborations are not always feasible or easy, however. Dance provides a significant challenge for science. Thriving on interaction, distributed and collective cognition and destabilization, dance offers a radically anti-reductionist approach to investigating the processes of cognition. At the same time, science poses significant challenges for dancemakers: How can the processes of dancemaking be described in ways that have utility beyond personal narrative? Can technology afford us a means of viewing brain processes *online*? In what ways will new scientific knowledge translate into viable dance pedagogy?

To address these issues, numerous independent and inter-dependent laboratories have sprung up, each supporting a variety of themes and topics. These span a wide range of implicit and explicit approaches[11] to dance cognition: neuroaesthetics (Cross and Ticini, 2012; Calvo-Merino et al. 2008), action observation (Calvo-Merino 2005; Jola, Ehrenberg and Reynolds 2012), kinesthetic empathy (Reynolds and Reason 2012; Paterson 2012), attention and attentional focus (Wulf 2007; Montero 2010), skill optimization (Bläsing et al. 2012), task-specific use of imagery in movement creation (May et al. 2012; Kirsh 2009; Barnard and deLahunta 2011), and the nature of the performative mind (Schmid 2013).[12]

Emerging research models include 'bi-directional' designs where neither dance nor science takes analytical primacy (Jola, Ehrenberg and Reynolds 2012: 22). Dancer-scientists work towards articulating flexible frameworks for understanding complex psychophysical dynamics (Bläsing et al. 2012). These researchers strive to capture inter-subjective experience (Gillespie and Cornish 2010; Barnard and deLahunta 2011) and avoid reducing embodiment to neural mechanisms. New methodologies are paving ways to span qualitative and quantitative distinctions in more creative ways (Berrol 2004; Gillespie and Cornish 2010; Gadamer 1998). Such new research initiatives have been successful not only in measuring outcomes in things in matters heretofore considered 'immeasurable' (Fortin 2005: 4), but also in generating more complex questions. Organizing and exploring 'improvisational, intuitive, and trial-and-error approaches' are achieving a greater dimension of ease while maintaining 'structured, systematic' (and 'therefore scientific') rigor (Jola 2010: 205).

New visual models, too, have been designed for understanding cognitive processes in dancemaking (Stevens et al. 2003; deLahunta, Clarke and Barnard 2012). Advances in neuro-imaging and neuro-behavioral studies have fostered our understanding of the 'dynamical coupling of brain, body, and environment' (Stafford, 2011: 31). As well, different empirical methods and tools of analysis are facilitating a better connection between lab and real-time experience (Stafford 2011: 2, 13). Small, but significant studies on action observation correlate brain data from imaging technology with subjective reporting on behavioral measures (May et al. 2012; Calvo-Merino et al. 2005; Cross et al. 2006; Jola, Ehrenberg and Reynolds 2012; Jola 2010).

Internet reportage

Internet sites have been vital sources for fostering dialogue, research analysis and networking around embodied cognition. Select sites serve as platforms for explication and discussion around the intersection of the arts (in general), science and design, with dance somewhat less represented than the other arts. Some of these sites are sponsored by a broad coalition of funders and include information-rich weblogs and other resources.

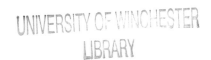

In the last decade a growing number of choreographers have sought to use publication – both traditional as well as digital – to disseminate their approaches to dancemaking. Some, but not all of these publication projects have included interdisciplinary dance-science research, but the objects they offer can be useful resources for this collaborative research. One example of a project that sought both to publish these unique objects as well as embrace interdisciplinary collaborative research was Motion Bank (www.motionbank.org) a four-year choreographic research project of The Forsythe Company. The main focus of the project is to build an archive of digital scores from guest choreographers. To date, scores include the works of William Forsythe, Deborah Hay, John Burrows, Matteo Fargion, Bebe Miller and Thomas Hauert. Running in parallel to the development of the on line scores was the Dance Engaging Science project funded by the Volkswagen Foundation that aimed to develop new collaborative research in the field of dance.

Another ambitious example of a social networking website employing a free-use platform is dance-tech.net (www.dance-tech.net). The thrust of this website is to explore new media and dialogue on innovative topics on embodiment involving the interplay of dance, science and digital media. Produced by Marlon Barrios Solano, dance-tech.net was launched in 2007 through multiple collaborations and networks across the United States of America and Europe. Dance-tech.net operates through a voluntary donation system, creative collaborations and bartering. Using digital technology creatively and expansively, dance-tech.net offers a platform for disseminating ideas and curating from a broad and inclusive perspective on embodied movement practices.[13] The website is designed to develop and maintain a broad series of online interdisciplinary workshops, interviews, pedagogical interventions and synergistic collaborations on a world scale. It entails a series of video interviews on different topics by artists, choreographers, researchers and theorists from the arts, science and humanities, arts administrators and producers, along with venues and technologies relevant to contemporary performance practices. At the time of this writing, more than 300 video programs have been produced and are available on the Internet for free viewing.

The Web also features sites on specialized topics within embodied cognition. One example is *Watching Dance* (http://www.watchingdance.org). *Watching Dance* focuses primarily on kinesthetic empathy and action observations, that is, how spectators respond to and identify with dance. Kinesthetic empathy is a multi-disciplinary study, including the fields of motor physiology and affective and social neuroscience With initial funding from the Arts and Humanities Research Council (2010–2011), *Watching Dance* continues to function as an active networking and discussion site, The website offers a range of resources including an interactive *Mind Map* that graphs multiple aspects of empathic communication.[14]

Challenges forward?

The road forward faces many challenges to organization, clarification and consolidation. Dancing clearly involves thinking, but dancemaking requires unique cognitive processes that demand deeper description and analysis (Stevens and McKechnie 2005; Hagendoorn 2010; Jola, 2010). Despite significant beginnings, research in cognition in dancemaking remains isolated and in need of greater global visibility and cohesion (deLahunta 2012). Creative clusters of thinkers and practitioners still need to advance theories and methods to evolve a focused discourse. Better access to resources and their utilization are needed, both within and outside of the academy.

International collaborators are enthusiastic and committed, benefiting from these collaborations in tangible and intangible ways (deLahunta, Barnard and McGregor 2009). Artistically, choreographers have reported gaining insights into their own processes, as well as inspiration into routes into new ways of starting, altering and elaborating on their usual processes of creating dance. The sciences have provided a new, experimental terrain for honing questions and hypotheses, as well as testing out new methodologies. Dancers have gained insights into their own processes, either uncovering different cognitive approaches or underscoring intuitive processes of improvisation and creativity and creativity (May et al. 2012).

These exchanges afford the opportunity to approach a single dance or choreographic problem within a dance from a range of perspectives. Paradigms for future multidisciplinary research across the arts and the sciences are emerging. Researchers are paving viable pathways towards understanding cognition in this context – or, rather, *host* of contexts. As each example of dancemaking is contextualized in its tasks and processes, its potential impact can be larger than the study parameters. Larger benefits to society depend on the sustainability of projects and their dissemination.

One of the largest barriers to the conversation remains the development of a shared, non-dualistic language or vocabulary for discourse (deLahunta 2013). What language best captures or describes the actual *experience* of dancing, either as performed or observed? What language is best suited to the lived experience of dance while building theoretical bridges to conceptual understanding and analysis? (Figure 1.2) The question of how to articulate a dance experience looms large within dance itself (Warburton 2011, Legrand and Ravn 2009; Roche 2011; Engel and Jeppesen 2010; Rouhiainen 2012). Through dance, the moving body becomes the link between thought and action, both intentionally and artistically. How can that embodied cognitive experience be captured in non-dualistic ways? (Sheets-Johnstone 2009; 2011b). The vocabulary should at the very least, preserve its unique integrity as a non-reductionist reality of the unity of body, brain and thinking (Sheets-Johnstone 2009). The problem is not only one of scientific reductionism, however. Dancers, too, are challenged to write *thick* descriptions of their experience. Despite a rich body of qualitative narrative from phenomenology and sociocultural studies, dance processes remain a-theoretical or 'under-theorized' (Rouhiainen 2012: 44). Terms used liberally in both disciplines merit clarification in light of synthetic research.

Further, the issue of dual competency also presents challenges. Dual competency is hard to come by. Each field should maintain its integrity (Klein 2007). Scientists themselves rarely participate in dancing *as* dancers, which makes it difficult to grasp the gestalt of the experience (Blumenfeld-Jones 2009). Dancers often desire, but lack the access to and the training in scientific procedures (Jola 2010; deLahunta, et al. 2012). Somatic psychologist Paul Vermersch suggests that this is a baseline to truly building a body of valid research that evades dualistic concepts of mind and body. To go…

> …beyond a naïve and uneducated use of introspection, and thus to enable it to become a research methodology, it seems to me that the minimum condition is first that it should be *effectively practised* by a community of researchers. This should take place over at least ten years or so, so that two or three successive research cycles (theses, publications, books) can begin to have cumulative effects, with each researcher having his own experience of introspection, and of guiding in an interview the introspection of other people.
>
> (Vermersch 2009: 27)

Current participants in the new dialogue foresee a time when cognitive neuroscience can embrace embodied cognition in dancemaking as living processes of movement (Sheets-Johnstone 2011; Legrand and Ravn 2009). Going forward means increasing specificity – the explicit characteristics (and their interactions) of the dancing body, the context, the choreographic rules employed, the working cognitive processes, the outcomes and the measuring tools. We have within our grasp the possibility of investigating the cognitive processes of dancemaking in ways where all parties have a voice (Reynolds, Jola, and Pollick, 2012; Borgdorff 2009; Jola 2010). Such interchanges are enabling dancers to assume more transmutable roles, such as dance teacher-scientist or dance artist-scientist (Galeota-Wozny 2011) with new forms and tools in and outside of the proverbial box (Dyer and Löytönen 2012). Time, patience and freedom to explore should go far toward sustaining the emergent knowledge.

Explorations for this chapter appear in Appendix II.

References

Bargh, J.A. (1994), 'The four horsemen of automaticity: Awareness, intention, efficiency, and control in social cognition', in R.S. Wyer, Jr. and T.K. Srull (eds.), *Handbook of Social Cognition* (2nd ed.). Hillsdale, NJ: Erlbaum, pp. 1–40.

Barnard, P., and deLahunta, S. (2011), 'Creativity and bridging', *Creative Research Center Blog Post*, Montclair State University, 19 April 2011. Accessed 31 December 2012.

Batson, G. (2013), 'Excribing the choreographic mind: Dance and neuroscience in collaboration', http://seadnetwork.wordpress.com/white-paper-abstracts/final-white-papers/ex-scribing-the-choreographic-mind-dance-neuroscience-in-collaboration/. Accessed 5 April 2014.

Berrol, C. (2004), 'The expanding options of experimental research design in dance/movement therapy', in R. Flaum Cruz and C. Berrol (eds.), *Dance/Movement Therapists in Action: A Working Guide to Research Actions*. Springfield, IL: Charles C. Thomas Publishers, pp. 23–44.

Birringer, J. and Fenger, J. (eds.) (2005), *Tanz im Kopf/Dance and Cognition*. Münster: LIT Verlag.

Bläsing, B., Calvo-Merino, B., Cross, E.S., Jola, C., Honisch, J. and Stevens, C.J. (2012), 'Neurocognitive control in dance perception and performance', *Acta Psychologica*, 139, pp. 300–08.

Bläsing, B., Puttke, M. and Schack, T. (eds.) (2010), *The Neurocognition of Dance: Mind, Movement and Motor Skills*. London: Routledge.

Blumenfeld-Jones, D. (2009), 'Bodily-kinesthetic intelligence and dance education: Critique, revision, and potentials for the democratic ideal', *The Journal of Aesthetic Education*, 43: 1, pp. 59–76.

Bohannon, J. (2008), 'Can scientists dance?', *Science*. 319: 5865, p. 905. http://www.sciencemag.org/content/319/5865/905.2.full. Accessed 29 December 2012.

Bohannon, J. (2011), 'A modest proposal', TedX-Brussels conference (http://www.ted.com/talks/john_bohannon_dance_vs_powerpoint_a_modest_proposal.html). Accessed 29 December 2012.

Borgdorff, H. (2009), *Artistic Research Within the Fields of Science*. Bergen, NW: Bergen Academy of Art and Design.

Borgdorff, H. (2006), 'The debate on research in the arts, http://www.gu.se/digitalAssets/1322/1322713_the_debate_on_research_in_the_arts.pdf. Accessed 20 August 2013.

Burns, S. (2007), 'Mapping Dance: Entrepreneurship and professional practice in dance higher education', *The Higher Education Academy*. Lancaster, UK: Palatine.

Burt, R. (2009), 'The specter of interdisciplinarity', *Dance Research Journal*, 41: 1. Online at http://muse.jhu.edu/journals/dance_research_journal/v041/41.1.burt.html. Accessed 4 August 2013.

Calvo-Merino, B., Glaser, D.E., Grèzes, J., Passingham, R.E. and Haggard, P. (2005), 'Action observation and acquired motor skills: An fMRI study with expert dancers', *Cerebral Cortex*, 15: 9, pp. 1243–49.

Calvo-Merino, B., Jola, C., Glaser, D.E. and Haggard, P. (2008), 'Towards a sensorimotor aesthetics of performing art', *Consciousness and Cognition*, 17: pp. 911–22.

Caspersen, D. (2011), 'Decreation: Fragmentation and unity', in S. Spier (ed.), *William Forsythe and the Practice of Choreography: It Starts From Any Point*. London: Routledge, pp. 93–100.

Cooper-Albright, A. (1997), *Choreographing Difference: The Body and Identity in Contemporary Dance*, Wesleyan University Press.

Cross, E.S., Hamilton, A.F.D.C., and Grafton, S.T. (2006), Building a motor simulation de novo: Observation of dance by dancers. *Neuroimage*, 31: 3, pp. 1257–67.

Cross, E.S. and Ticini, L.F. (2012), 'Neuroaesthetics and beyond: New horizons in applying the science of the brain to the art of dance', *Phenomenology and the Cognitive Sciences*, 11: 1, pp. 5–16.

Dale, J.A., Hyatt, J. and Hollerman, J. (2007), 'The neuroscience of dance and the dance of neuroscience: Defining a path of inquiry', *The Journal of Aesthetic Education*, 41: 3, pp. 89–110.

deLahunta, S. (2012), 'Dance engaging science', A proposal for a series of four workshops put forward to the Volkswagen Foundation by The Forsythe Company and The Department of Neurophysiology, Max Planck Institute for Brain Research, Frankfurt: (unpublished manuscript).

deLahunta, S., Barnard, P. and McGregor, W. (2009), 'Augmenting choreography: Using insights and inspiration from science', in J. Butterworth and L. Wildschut (eds.), *Contemporary Choreography: A Critical Reader*. New York: Routledge, pp. 431–48.

deLahunta, S. (2013), 'Publishing choreographic ideas', in E. Boxberger and G. Wittmann (eds.), *pARTnering Documentation: Approaching Dance, Heritage, Culture*. 3rd Dance Education Biennae 2012 Frankfurt am Main. Munchen, DE: Epodium Verlag, pp. 18–25.

deLahunta, S., Clarke, G. and Barnard, P. (2012), 'A conversation about choreographic thinking tools', *Journal of Dance & Somatic Practices*, 3: 1–2, pp. 243–59.

Dyer, B. and Löytönen, T. (2012), 'Engaging dialogue: co-creating communities of collaborative inquiry', *Research in Dance Education*, 13: 1, pp. 121–47.

Engel, L. and Jeppesen, R.S. (2010), 'The dance of words', *Nordic Journal of Dance*, 1, pp. 56–65.

Fortin, S. (2005), 'Measurable? Immeasurable? What are we looking for?', *Proceedings of the Laban Research Conference Day*. London: Laban Center, pp. 3–8.

Fraleigh, S. (1991), 'A vulnerable glance: Seeing dance through phenomenology', *Dance Faculty Publications*, Paper 4, The College of Brockport State University of New York, Digital Commons @ Brockport.

Gadamer, H-G. (1998), *Praise of Theory*. New Haven: Yale University Press.

Galeota-Wozny, N. (2011), formal interview by Batson, G., 18 October 2011.

Gehm, S., Husemann, P. and von Wilcke K. (eds.), *Knowledge in Motion: Perspectives of Artistic and Scientific Research in Dance,* New Brunswick, N.J.: Transaction Publishers.

Gillespie, A. and Cornish, F. (2010), 'Intersubjectivity: Towards a dialogical analysis', *Journal for the Theory of Social Behaviour*, 40: 1, pp. 19–46.

Grove, R., Stevens, C. and McKechnie. S. (eds.) (2005), *Thinking in Four Dimensions: Creativity and Cognition in Contemporary Dance*. Melbourne: Melbourne University Press.

Guertzkow, J. (2002), 'How the arts impact communities: An introduction to the literature on arts impact studies', Taking the Measure of Culture Conference July 7–8, Princeton University, Princeton, N.J.

Hagendoorn, I. (2010), 'Dance, language and the brain', *International Journal of Arts and Technology*, 3: 2, pp. 221–234.

Jola, C. (2010), 'Research and choreography: Merging dance and cognitive neuroscience', in B. Bläsing, M. Puttke and T. Schack (eds.), *The Neurocognition of Dance: Mind, Movement and Motor Skills*. London: Routledge, pp. 203–34.

Jola, C., Ehrenberg, S. and Reynolds, D. (2012), 'The experience of watching dance: Phenomenological–neuroscience duets', *Phenomenology and the Cognitive Sciences*, 11: pp. 17–37, published online.

Kirsh, D. (2009), 'Knowledge: Explicit vs. implicit', in T. Bayne, A. Cleeremans and P. Wilkine (eds.), *The Oxford Companion to Consciousness*. Cambridge: Oxford University Press, pp. 397–402.

Kirsh, D., et al. (2009), 'Choreographic methods for creating novel, high quality dance, Proceedings of the *5th International workshop on Design and Semantics of Form and Movement*, pp. 1880195. http://adrenaline.ucsd.edu/Kirsh/Articles/Interaction/kirshetal2009.pdf. Accessed 15 September 2013.

Klein, G. (2007), 'Dance in a knowledge society', in S. Gehm, P. Husemann and K. von Wilcke (eds.), *Knowledge in Motion: Perspectives of Artistic and Scientific Research in Dance*. Verlag: Transcripts, pp. 25–35.

Klein, J.T. (1990), *Interdisciplinarity: History, Theory, and Practice*. Detroit, IL: Wayne State University Press.

Kolcio, K. and Hingorani, M. (2011), 'Body languages: Contemporary biology', film http://www .youtube.com/watch?v=vZ6OTjMe1W8. Accessed 22 December 2012.

Kozel, S. (2007), *Closer: Performance, Technologies, Phenomenology*. Cambridge, MA: MIT Press.

Lansdale, J. (2005), 'Re-aligning dance research for the 21st century', in K. Vincs (ed.), *Dance Rebooted: Initializing the Grid*, Conference Proceedings, Ausdance National, December 2004, http://ausdance.org.au/publications/details/dance-rebooted-conference-papers. Accessed 5 April 2014.

Legrand, D. and Ravn, S. (2009), 'Perceiving subjectivity in bodily movement: The case of dancers', *Phenomenology and the Cognitive Sciences*, 8: 3, pp. 389–408.

Lepecki, A. (2004), *Of the Presence of the Body: Essays on Dance and Performance Theory*. Middletown, CT: Wesleyan University Press.

Lapuente, I. (2012), 'Co-creating cultures: Creation, change and transformation out of diversity', blogpost, http://co-creating-cultures.com/eng/?p=1727. Accessed 15 September 2013.

Liu, A. (2010), 'The elusive chimera: Interdisciplinary', online http://galeriaperdida.com/ andrealiu.pd. Accessed 19 September 2012.

Mason, P. (2009), 'Brain, dance and culture: Collaborative choreography and evolutionary characteristics in the work of Elizabeth Dalman', Brolga, online http://www.academia. edu/333198/Brain_Dance_and_Culture_2_Collaborative_choreography_and_evolutionary_ characteristics_in_the_work_of_Elizabeth_Dalman. Accessed 8 February 2013.

May, J., et al. (2012), 'Points in mental space: An interdisciplinary study of imagery in movement creation', *Dance Research Journal*, 29: 2, pp. 404–30.

McCarthy, R., Blackwell, A., deLahunta, S., Wing, A., et al. (2006), 'Bodies meet minds: Choreography and cognition, *Leonardo*, 39: 5, pp. 475–78.

Melrose, S. (2009), 'Visible thought: choreographic cognition in creating, performing, and watching contemporary dance', in J. Butterworth and L. Wildschut (eds.), *Contemporary Choreography: A Critical Reader*. New York: Routledge, pp. 23–37.

Miller, G.A. (2003), 'The cognitive revolution: A historical perspective', *Trends in Cognitive Sciences*, 7: 3, pp. 141– 4.

Mitchell, W. J., Inouye, A.S. and Blumenthal, M.S. (2003), *Beyond Productivity: Information, Technology, Innovation, and Creativity*. Washington, D. C.: National Academies Press.

Montero, B. (2010), 'Does bodily awareness interfere with highly skilled movement?', *Inquiry*, 53: 2, pp. 105–122.

Ostreng, W. (2010), *Science Without Boundaries: Interdisciplinarity in Research, Society, and Politics*. Lanham, MD: University Press of America.

Paterson, M. (2012), 'Movement for movement's sake? On the relationship between kinaesthesia and aesthetics', *Essays in Philosophy*, 13: 2, pp. 471–97.

Reid, T. (2011), 'Art-making and the arts in research universities', Prhtt//arts-u.org/wp-content/uploads/2012/03/ArtsEngine-National-Strategic-Task-Forces-Interim-Report-March-2012.pdf. Accessed 8 February 2013.

Reynolds, D. and Reason, M. (2012), *Kinesthetic Empathy in Creative and Cultural Contexts.* Bristol/Chicago: Intellect Books.

Reynolds, D., Jola, C. and Pollick, F.E. (2012), 'Editorial introduction & abstracts: Dance and neuroscience – New partnerships', *Dance Research*, 29, pp. 260–69.

Roche, J. (2011), 'Embodying multiplicity: the independent contemporary dancer's moving identity', *Research in Dance Education*, 12: 2, pp. 105–18.

Risner, D. (2012), 'Hybrid lives of teaching and artistry: A study of teaching artists in dance in the USA', *Research in Dance Education*, 13: 2, pp. 175–93.

Rouhiainen, L. (ed.) (2007), *Ways of Knowing in Dance and Art*, Volume 19, Acta Scenica. Helsinki:Theatre Academy.

Rouhiainen, L. (2012), 'An investigation into facilitating the work of the independent contemporary dancer through somatic psychology', *Journal of Dance & Somatic Practices*, 3: 1–2, pp. 43–59.

Schmid, W. (ed.) (2013), 'Performativity' in *The Living Handbook of Narratology*, http://hup.sub.uni-hamburg.de/lhn/index.php/Performativity. Accessed 12 February 2013.

Sheets-Johnstone, M. (ed.) (1992), *Giving the Body Its Due.* New York: SUNY Press.

Sheets-Johnstone, M. (2011), *The Primacy of Movement.* Amsterdam, NL: John Benjamins Publishers.

Sheets-Johnstone, M. (1981), 'Thinking in movement', *Journal of Aesthetics and Art Criticism,* 39: 4, pp. 399–07.

Sheets-Johnstone, M. (2009), *A Corporeal Turn: An Interdisiciplinary Reader.* Exeter, UK: Imprint Academic.

Stadler, Michael A. (1997), 'Distinguishing implicit and explicit learning', *Psychonomic Bulletin & Review,* 4: 1, pp. 56–62.

Stafford, B.M. (2011), *A Field Guide to the New Meta-Field.* Chicago, IL: University of Chicago Press.

Stevens, C. and McKechnie, S. (2005), 'Thinking in action: Thought made visible in contemporary dance', *Cognitive Processing*, 6: 4, pp 253–282.

Stevens, C., Malloch, S., McKechnie, S. and Steven, N. (2003), 'Choreographic cognition: The time-course and phenomenology of creating a dance', *Pragmatics & Cognition*, 11: 2, pp. 297–326.

Vermersch, P. (2009), 'Describing the process of introspection', *Journal of Consciousness Studies*, 16: 10–12, pp. 20–57.

Warburton, T. (2011), 'Of meanings and movements: Re-languaging embodiment in dance phenomenology and cognition', *Dance Research Journal*, 43: 2, pp. 65–83.

Wulf, G. (2007), *Attention and Motor Skill Learning.* Champaign, IL: Human Kinetics Press.

Notes

1 Mind mapping is a way of graphing multiple connections to a central idea. By drawing *branches* emanating from that central idea, you create a visual web of interrelated

concepts. The words act as images. They are more than synonyms; they suggest ways of depicting/representing knowledge in a more associative, rather than a linear, way. The concept of Mind Mapping was trademarked by Tony Buzan (1974), although the origins of the idea go way back in early civilization (http://www.mind-mapping.org/blog/mapping-history/roots-of-visual-mapping/). Mind mapping has been adapted for the current computer generation in a number of ways. For instructions, see https://mind42.com.

2   Sourcing implies the place where something begins. While the word originally referred to business strategizing, it has been adopted by dance artists to suggest an openness to expanding the context and content of dance by accessing globalized cultures of all kinds (http://ase.tufts.edu/drama-dance/dance/coursesDescriptions.asp). Through sourcing, solutions emerge out of a sphere of nested relationships and from the confluence of knowledge tributaries – physical and metaphysical, sociocultural, technological and teleological (Ostreng 2010).

3   Within the last few decades of the twentieth century, the amount of interchange between the arts, science and technology exceeded the amount of knowledge shared throughout the entire millennium (Klein 1990). Despite these initiatives, dance-science engagement remains under-represented in world knowledge cultures when compared with other crossover currents in art, science, engineering and technology sectors. Between 2009 and 2012, the publication *Leonardo* (the International Society for the Arts, Sciences and Technology) put out two international calls for submission of interdisciplinary curricula. Of the seventy courses received (largely from the United States of America, both undergraduate and graduate), none involved dance. (http://www.leonardo.info/index.htm). Select academic centers have profiled successful inter-disciplinary projects with dance the intellectual tether. Today, dance is a major hub of academic inter-disciplinarity, with Wesleyan University (USA) being a case in point, in which all majors offer a dance option within their curricula. http://www.wesleyan.edu/creativecampus/crossingdisciplines/index.html.

4   Dancemakers are entering into experiential and conceptual explorations around the inter-connections between embodied cognition and dancemaking. Suffice to say, though, that these exchanges/collaborations are neither solely initiated nor driven by cognitive neuroscientists nor by other members of the intelligentsia; rather, dancers and choreographers often generate these exchanges, seeking new ways to stimulate ideas and solve questions already set in motion by their movement creation and praxis in pursuit of 'new knowledge coming from embodied practice' (deLahunta 2013: 18).

5   See http://choreocog.net/papers.html for a sampling of papers and other materials relating to conferences and projects on cognitive neuroscience and dancemaking within the last decade, with particular emphasis on the art-science collaborations of choreographers Wayne McGregor and William Forsythe.

6   A clever example of this is John Bohannon's TED talks segment 'Dance vs. Powerpoint – A Modest Proposal' November 2011. Bohannon is a biologist, science journalist and dancer at Harvard University who runs an annual 'dance your Ph.D.' project (Bohannon 2008).

7   For a range of reports on select projects on embodied cognition, either artistic and/or scientific, visit:

http://synchronousobjects.osu.edu/
http://motionbank.org/en/William Forsythe
http://www.bbc.co.uk/news/health-17120495 Emily Cross
http://www.wellcome.ac.uk/stellent/groups/corporatesite/@msh_peda/documents/web_document/wtx050349.pdf
http://www.choreocog.net/ Wayne McGregor

8   Clearly, many independent dancers, philosophers, researchers and others also contributed their personal investigations and experiences on dance and cognition over the last two decades. Forsythe dancer Dana Caspersen's reflections (Caspersen 2011), constitutes one example. Independent dance researcher Ivar Hagendoorn published various articles on his website on cognitive neuroscience and dance (www.ivarhagendoorn.com). Cognitive psychologist Dr. Ruth Day (Duke University USA) and cognitive scientist Dr. David Kirsh (University of California San Diego, USA) have researched dance and cognition extensively. http://adrenaline.ucsd.edu/kirsh/.

9   One example is the multidisciplinary project *Watching Dance: Kinesthetic Empathy* funded by the Arts and Humanitites Research Council, UK. This project culminated in a conference in 2011, *Kinesthetic Empathy: Content and Context* (www.watchingdance.org), bringing together experts from neuroscience, dance, film, music, and contemporary embodied practices, to explore the nature and role of kinesthetic empathy. Another is the *Cognitive Futures in the Humanities* conference held in Bangor, Wales. http://www.bangor.ac.uk/cognitive-humanities/.

10   The term 'bi-directional' in the context of embodied cognition in dancemaking was identified first in an article by Jola, Ehrenberg and Reynolds (2012: 22), cited in the references.

11   Implicit vs. explicit research methodologies in part follow concepts of implicit and explicit learning in cognitive science/cognitive psychology. For explication, see Stadler 1997. More relevant, though, these terms relate to the measures used – implicit measures relating more to processes, while explicit measures relate to the products of task-based analysis. Measures of implicit cognition comprise a heterogeneous set of methods and procedures that differ from measures of explicit cognition by having at least one of the following characteristics: (a) reduced controllability; (b) lack of intention; (c) reduced awareness of the origins, meaning, or occurrence of a response; or (d) high efficiency of processing. See Bargh 1994; and Kirsh 2009.

12   The SEAD network (Science, Engineering, Art and Design) (http://seadnetwork.wordpress.com) has addressed challenges and opportunities facing these kinds of collaborations by soliciting from educators across these disciplines for papers. See Batson (2013), 'Ex-scribing the choreographic mind', the only submission on dance. http://seadnetwork.wordpress.com/white-paper-abstracts/final-white-papers/ex-scribing-the-choreographic-mind-dance-neuroscience-in-collaboration/.

13   One example of a broad-based platform was a three-week internet learning program piloted in the summer of 2013, called *Minded Motion*. This collaborative co-learning lab addressing the question: How can embodied knowledge be shared and deepened through the internet? What unique forms of collaborative learning and creative activity might

the internet offer? In the lab, Contact artist Nancy Stark Smith directed portions of her Underscore, an approach to improvisation that she has been developing for over 30 years. Over 60 participants from all over the world used these free internet-based tools to explore weekly questions – theoretically, experientially and reflectively - about embodiment, training and memory, composition, and politics of the body.

14 The Watching Dance mind map is located at http://www.watchingdance.org/Mind_Map/ Interactivemindmap/index.html.

Chapter 2

Locating the Discourse

As careful attention shows, thought itself is in an actual process of movement. That is to say, one can feel a sense of flow in the 'stream of consciousness' not dissimilar to the sense of flow in the movement of matter in general.

(David Bohm 1995 [1981]: ix)

Overview

The processes of making dance undoubtedly engage the whole of cognition: perception, attention, intuition, imagination, problem-solving, decision-making, memory and more. Embodied movement dynamics are outward signs of these cognitive processes. How can we study the implicit processes of dancemaking scientifically? How can we study these processes in situ without stripping the dance context of the richness of these dynamics? This chapter provides a historical snapshot of embodied cognitive theory and its relevance to dancemakers today.

Focusing in…

- How did embodiment theory arise within classical cognitive science?
- What relevance does this theory have for dance?
- What visual models or verbal descriptions capture dance cognition?
- Does dance afford scientists a more radical view of embodied cognition?

Experiential prelude

Can other art forms shed light on embodied cognitive processes? Take the following example from literature:

So then I as a contemporary creating composition in the beginning was groping toward a continuous present, a using everything a beginning again and again and then everything being alike then everything very simply everything was naturally simply different and so

I as a contemporary was creating everything being alike was creating everything naturally being naturally simply different, everything being alike.

(Gertrude Stein 1926: 101)

In what way(s) does this quote from Gertrude Stein resonate with your experience of dance, your grasp of thought processes, your understanding of thinking in dance?

Introduction

When the Centre George Pompidou (the 'Beaubourg')[1] opened in 1977, it stood as an architectural marvel – the façade a permanent scaffolding of colorful pipes, heating shafts and air ducts normally hidden from the naked eye. Unmasking the internal support system brought renewed appreciation of a metaphor of transmutable human design: the implicit rendered explicit – the inner mysteries of support revealed.

Biological movement – dynamical and expressive – is the outward and visible sign of inner mental or cognitive processes. These processes cannot be reduced to computations without losing the empathic meaning that emerges through spatiotemporal flow and changing dynamics. This implicit-to-explicit transmutation challenges science. How readily can contemporary science afford us a bridge between things seen and unseen? How readily can researchers capture something that 'won't stay still' (Sheets-Johnstone 2012a: 52)…that defies linguistic analysis? What vocabulary is compatible with dance experience? In the end, are we relegated only to the outcomes of these processes, or can the processes themselves be studied (Hutt 2010)?

Locating embodied cognition in dance is a place to start addressing these issues. How did embodied cognitive theory evolve? What is the scope of this theory? At this point in time, do dancemakers and cognitive neuroscientists have a mutually satisfying definition of embodied cognition? This chapter offers a brief overview of the history of cognitive science and the evolution of embodied cognitive theory. With dancemaking in mind, the chapter locates embodiment within two interrelated perspectives: the phenomenological and the neuro-phenomenological.

Cognition in dancemaking

Dancemaking is a process of transmission, transmutation and transformation (Bannon and Holt 2012; de Lima 2013). Dance arises from movement dynamics and communicates via empathic attunement. The transmission of both tangible and intangible dynamics occurs within both the dance collective as well as between dancers and audience. What is being transmitted and how? Generative and expressive, dance is a 'negotiation' of complex, ongoing movement happenings in a field of heightened sensory responsiveness. As Jonathan Burrows notes: 'Choreography is a negotiation with the patterns your body is thinking' (Burrows 2010: front piece).

Thinking and acting are linked inseparably in dance: thinking *in* action is thinking *as* action. Thought and movement are one. Movement and mind work reciprocally within explicit contexts to become the dance. As a communicative, body-based art, dance engages all of cognition: perception, attention, intention, intuition, decision-making, memory and more. But rather than arbitrarily segregating mental processes from the kinesthetic dynamics of movement, body- and mind-in-motion are conjoined by the intention to communicate through movement.

The difference for dance lies neither in any particular faculty of the brain nor cognitive process, but in the particulars of body use, which impact on the kinetics of thought. 'Communicative and expressive, [dance] is visual, spatial, temporal, kinesthetic, sensual, evocative, affective, dynamic, and rhythmic' (Stevens et al. 2003: 298). Cognitive processes in dancemaking call upon the rapid deployment of these (largely non-verbal) multimodal processes that are 'more hidden' (Glass and Stevens 2005). What the audience sees (and feels) is the energetic resonance from the ongoing display of 'kinetic tactile-kinesthetic body' dynamics unfolding in space and time (Sheets-Johnstone 2000: 343). These dynamics are integral to the lived experience of the dancer and his or her capabilities as a communicator (Fraleigh 1987). Dancers are invested deeply in the sensations of their physical bodies because these are the communicators. Both the experience and the projection of 'sensing-thinking while moving' convey meaning (Caspersen 2011: 94).

Dancemaking poses 'puzzles for the body to solve'. These 'puzzles' require dancers to 'cope'; that is, to enact answers through heightened kinesthetic and proprioceptive capacities in unusual and often challenging conditions (Noland 2009). Multi-system capabilities and capacities are engaged through collective problem-generating/solving through movement. Solutions emerge from harnessing physically resonant cooperation from dancing together (McKechnie and Stevens 2009). Dancers attend and attune to the immediacy of multiple bodies, mediating changing dynamics in space-time (Stevens and McKechnie 2005). Other bodies moving in the space with similar intent add to the generative power of problem-solving. In this way, dance has been described as 'distributed creativity' (Kirsh 2011).

Dance phenomenologist Maxine Sheets-Johnstone states that thinking is 'kinetic' (Sheets-Johnstone 2009: 30). She called dance cognition 'thinking in movement' (Sheets-Johnstone 1981; 2009: 34).[2] Sheets-Johnstone notes that thinking in movement is not the same as thinking of movement, the latter being an experience of 'discrete events' (Sheets-Johnstone 2011: 423). To the contrary, thinking in movement 'is not an assemblage of discrete gestures happening, one after the next, but an enfolding of all movement into a perpetually moving present' (Sheets-Johnstone 2011: 425). (Note how Gertrude Stein had a visceral understanding of this in her prose.) She describes dance as a 'dynamically-tethered thematic…[where] thinking in movement [is]…a perpetual dissolution and dilation, even a mutability, of here-now movements and a moving present' (Maxine Sheets-Johnstone 2009: 34). She states: 'thinking in [improvisational] movement' carries within it 'the dynamics of motion as they are unfolding in the movement – kinesthetically, kinematically, kinetically' (Sheets-Johnstone 2009: 35, 47).

The scholars cited above join a growing community of thinkers who assert that cognition is for action. "Cognition is of the body, arising from bodily experience (Sheets-Johnstone 2009; 2012) – that is, from movement. Dance cognition, then, is a 'kinetic bodily logos', a 'natural kinetic intelligence' steeped in phylogenetic history wherein 'intelligence in action is instinctive' and intuitive (Sheets-Johnstone 2011: 442, 424). A 'kinetic body logos' is the logic of 'sensory-space-time-force dynamics' (Sheets-Johnstone 2009: 33–34, 53). As such, thinking in movement (i.e., dancemaking) partakes of a 'nonlinguistic strata of experience' (Sheets-Johnstone 2011: 426). Thinking in movement is thinking in relational dynamics that develop 'outside of language' (2011: 433). Such thinking 'challenges our assumptions that all thinking is linked to language' or 'symbolic systems' (such as mathematics) (2011: 436). Sheets-Johnstone states:

> Thinking in movement is not the work of a symbol-making body, a body mediating its way through the world by means of a language…it is the work of an existentially resonant body…Such thinking is different 'not in degree', but in kind from thinking in words. Words are not sharper tools, but more precise instruments by which to think about dynamics, by which to hone our sense of space, time, energy, causality, or 'agentivity'.
>
> (2009: 47)

Many other dancemakers have concurred with Sheets-Johnstone on this (see, for example, Fraleigh 1987; Hanna 1987; de Lima 2013). Always in flux, dance experiences are hard to capture and describe in ways that can be repeated, generalized and shared (deLahunta 2013), precisely because they are non-linguistic. The experience is dynamic. By articulating experience verbally or in writing, its presence is altered (Noë 2012). Choreographers might write or create symbols or other written shorthand in creating dances. These 'scripts' or 'scores' serve as prompts, memory devices or springboards for problem-solving in choreographing (Dills 1998). As a graphic form of literacy, they are immediate, tactile and direct. These scripts/scores capture many aspects of movement that would require excessive written description to convey the details. Such cognitive prompts are not the actual material of dance, however (Louppe et al. 1994).[3] The 'score' may or may not be 'complete, coherent, consistent, with a start, an end and an intelligible process which links them at the level of events' (Vermersch 2009: 28–29). Verbal records, drawings, sketches or other materials are 'tool[s] for information, image and inspiration which acts as a source for what you will see, but whose shape may be very different from the final realization' (Burrows 2010: 141).

As a field embracing linguistics and phenomenology, cognitive science has subscribed to theories of embodied cognition since the 1970s. These theories are beginning to come to light within dance. What is the origin of embodied cognitive theory in science? What theories are finding resonance with dance studies? The following section locates embodied cognition as a relevant topic within dance studies. Included below is a brief overview of the history of cognitive science and a summary of the evolution of embodied cognitive theory. Dancemakers can broaden their perspectives on embodiment through consulting these scientific resources.

Cognitive science – a historical snapshot

The Stanford Encyclopedia defines human cognition as 'the brain's faculty for processing information and formulating knowledge' (Thagard 2010). Cognitive science (CS) is a relatively young science. Its roots can be traced back to the late nineteenth- and early twentieth-century philosopher/psychologists, including William James, Edmund Husserl and Franz Brentano,[4] men who developed scientific methods for studying conscious mental states.

In its short history, the field has burgeoned. Today, CS incorporates theories from multiple disciplines, including computer science, mathematics, phenomenology, artificial intelligence, robotics, linguistics and neuroscience. It would make sense that a field dedicated to defining the science of mind cannot survive uni-disciplinarity. To a large extent, CS has become inter-digitated with many branches of neuroscience and human movement studies (Figure 2.1). At the same time, it maintains claims to its independence as a distinct science with its own 'ontological commitment' (Shapiro 2010: 14).

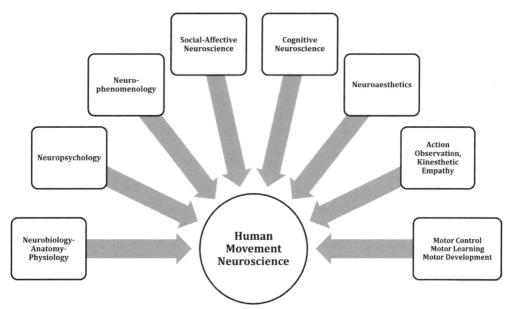

Figure 2.1: The evolving scope of human movement neuro-scientific studies.

The history of CS has undergone a number of revolutions in its brief history (Miller 2003; Gallagher and Zahavi 2012), from its formal inception in the 1950s through subsequent flowerings through the 1980s. This period also saw the impact of complexity science, dynamic systems-, chaos and non-linear theory on biology (Maturana and Varela 1980) as well as on CS (Van Orden and Stephen 2012). In the earliest phases of its history, CS largely adhered to computational and symbolic methods for explaining mental processes (Shapiro 2010; Stewart 2011). The brain was conceived of as a device that manipulated abstract symbols. Scientists viewed cognition primarily as a series of complex computations and symbol manipulations in the brain. Thought was of and in the brain, isolated from living, situated human experience. Thinking was the product of abstract neural symbols. Thought was an entity or 'mechanism' 'sandwiched between' sensory input and motor output (Stewart 2010: vii).

Since its formal founding, CS evolved three distinct periods: (1) computationalist (1950s–1970s) (Clark 1999; Miller 2003); (2) connectionist (neuronal network mapping integrated with dynamic systems theory) (1980s–1990s); and (3) second- into third-generation embodied or enactive cognition – that is, cognition as situated within lived experience (Shapiro 2010; Nagataki and Hirose 2007). These periods of development reflect in part historical tensions within positivism and materialism and other master discourses in twentieth-century postmodernism (Lyotard 1979; Rowlands 2010; Thagard 2012).

First-generation CS emerged as a reaction to behaviorism. Behaviorists proposed that the contexts of the brain could not be known. Classical (or standard) CS offered a fresh perspective in attempting to model the brain's contents and the components of mind (Albright, Kandel and Posner 2000). At the same time, standard CS evolved with 'a lingering division between the subjective mind and the objective body, the one only accessible from within, or from the so-called first-person perspective, the other only accessible from without, or from a third-person perspective…' (Fuchs 2011: 198). Further, as brain and nervous system assumed the privileged position in cognition (top-down processing of higher levels of cognition in theory of mind), the body's role (and more importantly, bodily movement) was relegated to a lower level of importance in cognitive modeling (Lakoff and Johnson 1980; 1999).

For the first four decades of the history of CS, abstract renderings were designed to capture the complexity of mental activity. These were based largely on computer models of search, match, retrieve, deduce etc. (Anderson 2003). These evolved into descriptions of mental states (perception, attention-intention, decision-making, judging, reflecting, memory and recall, language formation and semantics and other capacities) (Neisser 1967; Albright, Kandel and Posner 2000). From the 1960s through the 1980s, the activities and goals of CS aimed to map the brain's ultrastructure and detail its implicit contents (Shapiro 2010: 14; Clark 1999).

Mathematical and computational models still hold primacy in understanding how the brain 'represents' mental events (Johnson 2008: 159), and how mind evolves from neural schemas (Carrington and Bailey 2008; Gallese and Goldman 1998; Goldman and deVignemont 2009). Resistance to the idea of bodily consciousness stymied the advancement of any coherent theory of embodied cognition (Gallagher and Zahavi 2012; Shapiro 2010). For example, perception was categorized as a sensory 'module' or 'mechanism', one step along the linear sequential construction of cognition (Stewart 2010: vii). The perceiver's experience was not considered instrumental in the formation of cognition (Gallagher and Zahavi 2012).

According to Shaun Gallagher and Dan Zahavi (2012), five major movements within CS helped advance a scientific concept of embodied cognition:

1. The overall relaxation of the positivist research climate (Gallagher and Zahavi 2012) and the recognition of the benefits of interdisciplinary research (Ostreng 2009). Concurrent with the easing of the research climate was the phenomenal growth of pan-scholarly discourse around the self and embodiment. These concepts assumed center stage throughout the postmodern period (Bresler 2004; Hendrickson and McKelvey 2002).[5]
2. A focused direction within CS on advancing a scientific methodology for the study of consciousness. This direction helped forge alliances between CS and phenomenology in understanding the nature of experience (Chalmers 1995; Johnson 2008; Gallagher and Zahavi 2012).
3. The evolution of complexity theory, dynamic systems theory, ecological psychology and learning and developmental theories. Cognition is now viewed as the 'dynamical coupling of brain, body, and environment' (Stafford 2011: 31), a co-creation rather than a function of isolated neural processes (Varela, Thompson and Rosch 1991; Clark 1997). Scientists began to support the notion that embodiment is the integrated functioning of body, mind and context (Varela, Thompson and Rosch 1991). The brain evolved because of and for movement (Sheets-Johnstone 2009; Berthoz 2000; Doidge 2007; Noë 2007; Damasio 2012). Scientists advanced a methodology for the study of personal consciousness (Varela 1999; Petitmengin 2009; Thompson 2001 and 2007). This model previewed a scientifically rigorous approach to studying first-person experience and inter-subjectivity (Thompson 2001).
5. The flurry of discoveries within neuroscience and brain-mapping (imaging) technology throughout the 1990s. This- and other technological advancements brought online visibility to brain processes. American President George H. Bush dubbed the 1990s 'the decade of the brain' (Tandon 2000: 199) because of the volume of neurological discoveries. This decade was followed by the 'decade of the mind' (Olds 2011). Discoveries in brain-mapping (imaging) research advanced theories on neuroplasticity and the mirror neuron system. Other technological and behavioral advances enabled investigation for the first time into the inner workings of the self and inter-subjectivity, bringing neuroscience to the forefront of intellectual discussions on embodiment.

The embodiment hypothesis

Alternative arguments and models to classical CS began to appear in the 1970s (Dreyfus 1972; Varela 1977). This intellectual climate gave strength to the idea of cognition as an empirical science. A new breed of thinkers began to speculate, quite radically at the time, that thought did not arise exclusively in the brain. For them, cognition was seen to arise out of the body – actively moving in its context. Cognition, then, is for action, deeply situated and constrained by real-time demands (Wilson 2002). That cognition is contextual means that cognition is not only of the body (i.e., embodied). Cognition also is embedded and enmeshed in its context, extended through imagination and technology (Gallagher 2004), enacted through agency (Stewart 2010; Varela, Thompson and Rosch 1991) and empathic (endowed with resonant communication) (Reynolds and Reason 2012).

Between the 1970s and the 1990s, cognitive scientists aligned themselves with phenomenology, carving a niche for embodiment (Lakoff and Johnson 1999). CS partook of seminal works in phenomenology, psychology and humanism through the writings of Heidegger, Piaget, Vygotsky, Merleau-Ponty, Dewey and others. These works helped entrench phenomenological foundations for cognition within CS (Anderson 2003; Johnson 2008). Phenomenological embodiment played a vital role in advancing the understanding of the role of experience in learning and meaning (Johnson 2008).[6] To embrace phenomenology within CS meant 'giving the body its due' (Sheets-Johnstone 1992). Human organisms were viewed as constructions, a 'meshwork of selfless selves' (Varela 1991: 79), whose thoughts and actions could not be reduced to a single process (Stewart, Gapenne and DiPaolo 2010).

Embodied cognition and the neuro-phenomenological proposition

A pivotal figure in the embodiment movement within CS was Chilean biologist (and later, cognitive neuroscientist) Francisco Varela (1946–2001). Varela advocated a more embodied approach to cognition as early as the late 1960s and early 1970s. He conceived of the mind as fundamentally inseparable from subjective experience, its biological embodiment and its situated context in the world (Rudrauf et al. 2003). Varela was also a Buddhist. It was through his deep understanding of science combined with his practice of Buddhism that he arrived at key insights into first-person methodology in science. Following the ideas of Husserl and Merleau-Ponty, Varela worked out a radical 'neuro-phenomenology' of embodied thought (Varela 1996: 330). Concurring with the ideas of Heidegger, Varela believed that phenomenology was not a passive study; one must do phenomenology.[7] Phenomenology is 'empirical'. It is 'self-investigation evolving out of interaction and relationships with others, lived and reflected upon' (Ihde 2012: 3, 6).

By the 1990s, Varela coined the term 'embodied cognition' and conceptually framed its theories (Varela, Thompson and Rosch 1991). 'Embodied cognition' placed the biological and contextual body squarely in the center of the debate on consciousness and cognition (Varela,

Thompson and Rosch 1991). From this perspective, the brain is comprised of the dynamics of interaction – 'the plastic, non-localized processual nature of the moving consciousness' (Fuchs 2011: 196). Thought is co-generated from the biological body's capacities in living relationship to its environmental context. Cognition, then, was the product of 'embodied action' (Varela, Thompson and Rosch 1991: 172). Experience resulted from '...having a body with various sensorimotor capacities and that these individual sensorimotor capacities are themselves embedded in a more encompassing biological, psychological, and cultural context' (Clark 1999).

Proposed as an alternative to dualistic divisions between the mental and the physical, embodied cognition offered a window of transparency between the objective (outwardly perceived) and the subjective (and inter-subjective) body (Fuchs 2009). Embodiment theory prefaced the importance of autonomy and intentionality (Maturana and Varela 1980) as well as the intimate coupling of perception–action expounded by ecological psychologist J.J. Gibson (Gibson 1979). Here, humans are autonomous agents with exquisitely tuned sensory systems. Attunement links perceiver, environment and task. For Varela and his descendants, embodiment did not mean merely having a body, but also engaging with the world through active bodily awareness and attunement as a chief resource in engaging as a living system: not in isolation, but always in relationship (Weber and Varela 2002: 117). This coupling of living organism (system) and world is always relational; an interface indispensible for the acquisition [and meaning] of knowledge (Colombetti 2010: 149). The coupling is embodied and 'inseparable from and shaped by the concrete extra-cerebral structures and dynamics of the body and the body's embeddedness in the natural and social world' (Morris 2010: 235). Perception is not one step in a linear process of brain computations toward thinking and acting; rather, perception is the reality itself, wedded inextricably to action (Noë 2012). These debates emerged concurrently with the cresting praxis dialogue between postmodern dance and the Somatics movement.

Within CS, embodiment posed a significant challenge to traditional theory by placing bodily experience in the center of knowledge, and causal to cognition. Embodiment posed challenges to those adhering to information-science models (Tschacher and Bergomi 2011). In resolving the problem of the dualist 'inside/outside' debate of brain and world, questions needed to be posed within the framework of self-regulatory dynamics. Rather than, 'Do the neural processes of cognition extend beyond the brain?', the question could be reconceptualized and restated as: 'How must a system be organized in order to operate autonomously?' (Thompson and Stapleton 2008: 23–24).

Emerging theories around embodied cognition reflected closer theoretical and methodological cooperation between psychology, neuroscience, phenomenology and a variety of other fields that focus on the value interplay between perception, cognition and the environment (Albright, Kandel and Posner 2000). The enthusiastic embrace of these ideas signaled an important shift away from the isolationist view of the human brain/ mind, distanced from human experience. Such interactions enabled scientists to grasp how contextualized bodily experience might give rise to thought (Damasio 1999).

Three generations of researchers passed before CS formally adopted the embodiment hypothesis (Varela 1984; Varela, Thompson and Rosch 1991; Shapiro 2010; Nagataki and Hirose 2007). In introducing a 'science of experience' into CS, embodied cognition helped forge a more radical framework around the question of what constitutes data or evidence (Ihde 2012: 9). Today, phenomenology has become inextricably linked with cognitive neuroscience. A neuro-phenomenological synthesis shows promise as a foundational rubric for evolving a methodology for studying embodied cognition (Gallagher and Zahavi 2012; Varela 1996).

Despite shifts within traditional theory, embodied cognition remains a hotly debated topic (Adams 2010; Aizawa 2007; Chemero 2009; Dennett 1991; 2001; 2007). Embodied cognition is not one theory, but many theories (Gallagher 2000; Rowlands 2010; Shapiro 2010). As such, it is considered more akin to a set of research programs rather than a fully tested theory (Shapiro 2010). The degree to which the body is foregrounded in the formation of thought varies widely among investigators. Speculations run the gamut from the most conservative perspective in which the body merely is involved in the formation of thought, to more radical or dynamic theories in which the body is constitutive of thought.

Getting somewhere

The alignment of CS with phenomenology led to a significant shift within the science of mind. Interdisciplinary research on embodiment afforded more compatible ground on which to converse. Yet, praxis-based and praxis-driven research is not universal nor does it transcend disciplinarity. Therefore, in building an empirical science of embodied cognition within dance, movement creation and praxis must be the foundation. In this respect, dance scholars argue that cognitive neuroscience does not go far enough in embracing movement as primal (Sheets-Johnstone 2011; 2009; deLahunta 2013).

Movement is an affront to any Cartesian view of cognition. For dancemaking, it is neither the body in any particular feature, faculty or role, nor state of embodiment that is the root of thinking, but rather animate movement with its processual dynamics (Sheets-Johnstone 2009; 2011). Movement deposes the brain from a privileged position of being the chief executive officer toward foregrounding movement as vital in co-creating thought and action (Sheets-Johnstone 2011; 2012a; 2012b; Fuchs 2011). Throughout evolution and development, the primacy of movement is essential to the formation of thought – a notion that remains radical (Sheets-Johnstone 2011).

Collaborations between dancers and scientists are helping to model embodied cognition in dance. It is an exciting moment of commitment to understanding dance praxis within science. Today, embodied cognition is becoming more theoretically complex (Wilson and Foglia 2011). This keeps the discussion lively. Our understanding of implicit processes is now grasped through a variety of digital media, technologies and behavioral measures.

These capture the dynamics of movement at increasingly sophisticated scales of analysis. These technologies are young, and while valuable, pose limitations to answering questions adequately about embodied cognition (Witowski 2011) and about embodied cognition within dancemaking (Jola 2010; May et al. 2012).

Finally, it bears restating that one important need is to evolve a shared, non-dualist vocabulary that communicates to all parties (Barnard and deLahunta 2011). This is as much a charge for dance, as it is for science. Articulating the fullness and complexity of dance experience remains a priority (Warburton 2011; Sheets-Johnstone 2009; Rouhiainen 2012). The 'relatively unarticulated terrain of dance might cloud the clarity of our understanding of research and lead us to assume that anything articulate about dance is research' (Bannerman 2009: 234). The complex abstractedness of science also needs to be bridged. We can open to many rationalities and multi-logics in the quest for interconnectedness and interrelatedness. At the same time, our differences constitute vital 'points of tension' that both challenge us and offer us a means forward (Bannerman 2009: 232).

Bridges are forming (deLahunta, Barnard and McGregor 2009). We can proceed at once passionately yet cautiously, as we cobble together new relationships in the spirit of the 'bricoleur' (Kincheloe 2001; Bales 2008). As we continue to dialogue within the sphere of embodiment, we are reminded of the words of phenomenologist Maurice Merleau-Ponty, who said: 'movement must somehow cease to be a way of designating things or thoughts, not its clothing but its token or its body' (Merleau-Ponty 1962: 182).

Explorations for this chapter appear in Appendix II.

References

Adams, F. (2010), 'Embodied cognition', *Phenomenology and the Cognitive Sciences*, 9: 4, pp. 619–28.

Aizawa, K. (2007), 'Understanding the Embodiment of Perception', *Journal of Philosophy*, 104: 1, pp. 5–25.

Albright, T., Kandel, E. and Posner, M. (2000), 'Cognitive neuroscience', *Current Opinion in Neurobiology*, 10: 5, pp. 612–24.

Anderson, M. (2003), 'Embodied cognition: A field guide', *Artificial Intelligence*, 149: 1, pp. 91–130.

Bales, M. (2008), 'A dancing dialectic', in M. Bales and R. Nettl-Fiol (eds.), *The Body Eclectic: Evolving Practices in Dance Training*, Chicago, IL: University of Illinois Press, pp. 10–21.

Bannerman, C. (2009), 'Viewing a/new: The landscape of dance in 2009', *Research in Dance Education*, 10: 3, pp. 231–40.

Bannon, F., and Holt, D. (2013), 'Touch: Experience and knowledge', *Journal of Dance and Somatic Practices*, 3: 1, pp. 215–27.

Barnard, P. and deLahunta, S. (2013), 'Creativity and Bridging'. Blogpost 19 April 2011. Creative Research Center, Montclair State University. https://blogs.montclair.edu/

creativeresearch/2011/04/19/creativity-and-bridging-by-philip-barnard-and-scott-delahunta/. Accessed 29 August 2013.

Bateson, G. (1979), *Mind in Nature: A Necessary Unity*, New York, NY: E.P. Dutton.

Bermudez, L. (2003), *Thinking Without Words*, Oxford: Oxford University Press.

Berthoz, A. (2000), *The Brain's Sense of Movement*, Cambridge, MA: Harvard University Press.

Bläsing, B., Puttke, M. and Schack, T. (eds.) (2010), *The Neurocognition of Dance: Mind, Movement and Motor Skills*, London: Routledge.

Bohm, D. (1995 [1981]), *Wholeness and the Implicate Order*, London: Routledge.

Bresler, L. (2004), *Knowing Bodies, Moving Minds: Towards Embodied Teaching and Learning*, London: Kluwer Academic Publishers.

Burrows, J. (2010), *A Choreographer's Handbook*, Milton Park, Abingdon, Oxon; New York, NY: Routledge.

Carrington, S. and Bailey, A. (2008), 'Are there theory of mind regions in the brain? A review of the neuroimaging literature', *Human Brain Mapping*, 30: 8, pp. 2313–35.

Caspersen, D. (2011), 'Decreation: Fragmentation and unity', in S. Spier (ed.), *William Forsythe and the Practice of Choreography: It Starts From Any Point*, London: Routledge, pp. 93–100.

Chalmers, D. (1995), 'Facing up to the problem of consciousness', *Journal of Consciousness Studies*, 2: 3, pp. 200–19.

Chemero, A. (2009), *Radical Embodied Cognitive Science*, Cambridge, MA: MIT Press.

Clark, A. (1997), *Being There: Putting Brain, Body, and World Together Again*, Cambridge MA: MIT Press.

——— (1999), 'An embodied cognitive science?', *Trends in the Cognitive Sciences*, 3: 9, pp. 345–51.

Colombetti, G. (2010), 'Enaction, sense-making and emotion', in J. Stewart, O. Gapenne, E. Di Paolo (eds.), *Enaction: Towards a New Paradigm for Cognitive Science*, Cambridge, MA: MIT Press.

Damasio, A. (2012), *Self Comes to Mind: Constructing the Conscious Brain*, New York, NY: Vintage Books.

——— (1999), *The Feeling of what Happens: Body and Emotion in the Making of Consciousness*, New York, NY: Harcourt Brace.

Davidson, A. (2013), 'Somatics: An orchid in the land of technology', *Journal of Dance and Somatic Practices*, 5: 1, pp. 3–15.

deLahunta, S. (2013), 'Publishing choreographic ideas', in Boxberger, E. and Wittmann, G. (eds.), *pARTnering Documentation: Approaching Dance, Heritage, Culture.* 3rd Dance Education Biennae 2012 Frankfurt am Main. Munchen, DE: Epodium Verlag, pp. 18–25.

———, Barnard, P. and McGregor, W. (2009), 'Augmenting choreography: Insights and inspiration from science', in J. Butterworth, and L. Wildschut (eds.), *Contemporary Choreography: A Critical Reader*, New York, NY: Routledge, pp. 431–48.

de Lima, C. (2013), 'Trans-meaning – Dance as an embodied technology of perception', *Journal of Dance and Somatic Practices*, 5: 1, pp. 17–30.

Dennett, D. (1991), *Consciousness Explained*, Boston: Little, Brown and Co.

—— (1993), 'Review of F. Varela, E. Thompson and E. Rosch, The Embodied Mind', *American Journal of Psychology*, 106, pp. 121–26. http://ase.tufts.edu/cogstud/papers/varela.htm. Accessed 14 February 2013.

—— (2001), 'Are we explaining consciousness yet?', *Cognition*, 79: 1, pp. 221–37.

—— (2007), 'Heterophenomenology reconsidered', *Phenomenology and the Cognitive Sciences*, 6: 1–2, pp. 247–70.

Dills, A. (1998), 'Capturing dance on paper', *The Journal of Physical Education, Recreation and Dance*, 69: 6, pp. 27–31.

Doidge, N. (2008), *The Brain that Changes Itself*, New York, NY: Viking.

Dreyfus, H. (1972), *What Computers Can't Do: A Critique of Artificial Reason*, New York, NY: Harper & Row.

Forte, M. and Bonini, E. (2010), 'Embodiment and enaction: Theoretical overview for cybercommunities', in M. Iaonnides et al. (eds.), *Heritage in the Digital Era*, Paris: C2RMF, http://www.academia.edu/203784/EMBODIMENT_AND_ENACTION_A_THEORETICAL_OVERVIEW_FOR_CYBERCOMMUNITIES. Accessed 22 September 2013.

Fraleigh, S.H. (1987), *Dance and the Lived Body: A Descriptive Aesthetics*, Pittsburgh, PA: University of Pittsburgh Press.

Fuchs, T. (2011), 'The brain – A mediating organ', *Journal of Consciousness Studies*, 18: 7–8, pp. 196–221.

—— and De Jaegher, H. (2009), 'Enactive intersubjectivity: Participatory sense-making and mutual incorporation', *Phenomenology and Cognitive Science*, 8, pp. 465–86.

Gallagher, S. and Zahavi, D. (2012), *The Phenomenological Mind*, 2nd edn, New York, NY: Routledge.

Gallagher, S. (2004), 'Hermeneutics and the cognitive sciences', *Journal of Consciousness Studies*, 11: 10–11, pp. 162–74.

—— (2000), 'Philosophical conceptions of the self: Implications for cognitive science', *Trends in the Cognitive Sciences*, 4: 1, pp. 14–21.

Gallese, V. and Goldman, G. (1998), 'Mirror Neurons and the simulation theory of mind reading', *Trends in the Cognitive Sciences*, 2: 12, pp. 493–501.

Gibson, J. (1979), *The Ecological Approach to Visual Perception*, Boston: Houghton Mifflin.

Glass, R. and Stevens, C. (2005), 'Making sense of contemporary dance: An Australian investigation into audience interpretation and enjoyment levels', Short Report Prepared for *fuel4arts*, February 2005 MARCS Auditory Laboratories & School of Psychology University of Western Sydney.

Goldman, A. and deVignemont, F. (2009), 'Is social cognition embodied?', *Trends in the Cognitive Sciences*, 13: 4 154–59.

Hanna, J.L. (1987), *To Dance is Human: A Theory of Non-Verbal Communication*, Chicago, IL: University of Chicago Press.

Heidegger, M. (2000), *Introduction to Metaphysics*, New Haven, CT: Yale University Press.

Henrickson, L. and McKelvey, B. (2002), 'Foundations of "new" social science: Institutional legitimacy from philosophy, complexity science, postmodernism, and agent-based modeling', *Proceedings of the National Academy of Sciences of the United States of America*, 99: 3, pp. 7288–95.

Hutt, K. (2010), 'Corrective alignment and injury prevention strategies; Science, Somatics or both?', *Journal of Dance & Somatic Practices*, 2: 2, pp. 251–63.

Ihde, D. (2012), 'Can continental philosophy deal with the new technologies?', *The Journal of Speculative Philosophy*, 26: 2, pp. 321–32.

Jola, C. (2011), 'The experience of watching dance: Phenomenological – neuroscience duets', http://unicog.academia.edu/CorinneJola. Accessed 5 August 2013.

Johnson, M. (2008), *The Meaning of the Body*, Chicago: University of Chicago Press.

Jola, C. (2010). 'Research and choreography', in B. Bläsing, M. Puttke and T. Schack (eds.), *The Neurocognition of Dance: Mind, Movement and Motor Skills*, New York, NY: Psychology Press.

Kincheloe, J. (2001), 'Describing the bricolage: Conceptualizing a new rigor in qualitative research', *Qualitative Inquiry*, 7: 6, pp. 679–92.

Kirsh, D., Muntanyola, D., Jao, R.J., Lew, A. and Sugihara, M. (2009), 'Choreographic methods for creating novel, high-quality dance', *Design and Semantics of Form and Movement*, http://adrenaline.ucsd.edu/Kirsh/publications.html. Accessed 14 February 2013.

Lakoff, G. and Johnson, M. (1980), *Metaphors We Live By*, Chicago, IL: University of Chicago Press.

—— (1999), *Philosophy in the Flesh: The Embodied Mind and Its Challenge to Western Thought*, New York, NY: Basic Books.

Louppe, L. (ed.) (1994), *Traces of Dance: Drawings and Notations of Choreographers*, Paris: Editions Dis Voi.

Lyotard, J.-F. (1979), *The Postmodern Condition: A Report on Knowledge*, G. Bennington and B. Massumi (trans.), Manchester, UK: Manchester University Press.

May, J., Calvo-Merino, B., deLahunta, S., McGregor, W, Cusack, R., Owen, A. and Barnard, P. (2011), 'Points in mental space: An interdisciplinary study of imagery in movement creation', *Dance Research*, 29: 2, pp. 402–30.

McKechnie, S. and Stevens, C.J. (2009), 'Visible thought: Choreographic cognition in creating, performing, and watching contemporary dance', in J. Butterworth and L. Wildschut (eds.), *Contemporary Choreography*, London: Routledge, pp. 38–51.

Maturana, H. and Varela, F. (1973/1980), *Autopoiesis and Cognition: The Realization of the Living*, London: Riedl.

Merleau-Ponty, M. (1962), *Phenomenology of Perception*, London: Routledge

Miller, G.A. (2003), 'The cognitive revolution: A historical perspective', *Trends in Cognitive Sciences*, 7: 3, pp. 141–44.

Morris, D. (2010), 'Empirical and phenomenological studies of embodied cognition', *Handbook of Phenomenology and Cognitive Science*, Netherlands: Springer, pp. 235–52.

Nagataki, S. and Hirose, S. (2007), 'Phenomenology and the third generation of cognitive science: Towards a cognitive phenomenology of the body', *Human Studies*, 30: 3, pp. 219–32.

Nagel, T. (1974), 'What is it like to be a bat?', *The Philosophical Review*, 83: 4, pp. 435–50.

Noë, A. (2007), 'Making worlds available', in S. Gehm, P. Husemann and K. von Wilcke (eds.), *Knowledge in Motion: Perspectives of Artistic and Scientific Research in Dance*, New Brunswick, NJ: Transaction Publishers, pp. 121–28.

Noë, A. (2012), *Varieties of Presence*, Cambridge, MA: Harvard University Press.

Neisser, U. (1967*), Cognitive Psychology*, New York, NY: Appleton-Century-Crofts.

Noland, C. (2009), *Agency and Embodiment: Performing Gestures/Producing Culture*, Cambridge, MA: Harvard University Press.

Olds, J. (2011), 'For an international decade of the mind', *Malaysian Journal of Medical Science*, 18: 2, pp. 1–2.

Ostreng, W. (2009), *Science Without Boundaries: Interdisciplinarity in Research, Society and Politics*, Blue Ridge Summit, PA: University Press of America.

Petitmengin, C. (2009), 'The validity of first-person descriptions as authenticity and coherence', *Journal of Consciousness Studies*, 16: 10–12, pp. 252–84.

Reynolds, D. and Reason, M. (2012), *Kinesthetic Empathy in Creative and Cultural Contexts*, Bristol/Chicago: Intellect Books.

Rouhiainen, L. (2012), 'An investigation into facilitating the work of the independent contemporary dancer through somatic psychology', *Journal of Dance and Somatic Practices*, 3: 1 and 2, pp. 43–59.

Rowlands, M. (2010), *The New Science of the Mind*, Cambridge MA: MIT Press.

Rudrauf, D., Lutz, A., Cosmelli, D., Lachaux, J. and Le Van Ouven, M. (2003), 'From autopoiesis to neurophenomenology: Francisco Varela's exploration of the biophysics of being', *Biological Research*, 36: 1, pp. 27–65.

Shapiro, L. (2010), *Embodied Cognition*, New York, NY: Routledge.

——— (2010b), 'James Bond and the barking dog: Evolution and extended cognition', *Philosophy of Science*, 77: 3, pp. 400–18.

Sheets-Johnstone, M. (1981), 'Thinking in movement', *The Journal of Aesthetics and Art Criticism*, 39: 4, pp. 399–407.

——— (1992), *Giving the Body its Due*, New York, NY: SUNY Press.

——— (2000), 'Kinetic Tactile-Kinesthetic Bodies: Ontogenetical Foundations of Apprenticeship Learning', *Human Studies*, 23: 4, pp. 343–70.

——— (2009), *The Corporeal Turn: An Interdisciplinary Reader*, Exeter, UK: Imprint Academic.

——— (2011), *The Primacy of Movement*, expanded 2nd edn, Philadelphia: John Benjamin Publishing Company.

——— (2012a), 'From movement to dance', *Phenomenology and the Cognitive Sciences*, 11: 1, pp. 39–57.

——— (2012b), 'Movement and mirror neurons: A challenging and choice conversation', *Phenomenology and the Cognitive Sciences*, 11: 3, pp. 385–401.

Stark-Smith, N. (1982), 'Dance in translation: The hieroglyphs', *Contact Quarterly*, 7: 2, pp. 43–46.

Stein, G. (1926), *Composition as Explanation*, London: L. & V. Woolf at the Hogarth Press.

Stevens, C., Malloch, S., McKechnie, S. and Steven, N. (2003), 'Choreographic cognition: The time-course and phenomenology of creating a dance', *Pragmatics and Cognition*, 11: 2, pp. 297–326.

Stevens, C. and McKechnie, S. (2005), 'Thinking in action: Thought made visible in contemporary dance', *Cognitive Processing*, 6: 4, pp. 243–52.

Stewart, J. (2011), 'Foundational issues in enaction as a paradigm for cognitive science: From the origin of life to consciousness and writing', in J. Stewart, O. Gapenne and E.A. Di Paolo (eds.), *Enaction: Toward a New Paradigm for Cognitive Science*, London: MIT Press.

Stewart, J., Gapenne, O. and Di Paolo, E.A. (eds.) (2011), *Enaction: Toward a New Paradigm for Cognitive Science*, London: MIT Press.

Tandon, P. (2000), 'The decade of the brain: A brief review', *Neurology India*, 48: 3, pp. 199–207.

Thagard, P. (2010), 'Cognitive science', *Stanford Encyclopedia of Philosophy*. http://plato.stanford.edu/entries/cognitive-science/. Accessed 11 October 2012.

Thelen, E. and Smith, L. (1996), *A Dynamic Systems Approach to the Development of Cognition and Action*, Cambridge, MA: MIT Press.

Thompson, E.T. (ed.) (2001), *Between Ourselves: Second-Person Approaches to the Study of Consciousness*, Charlottesville, VA: Imprint Academic.

Thompson, E. (2007), *Mind in Life: Biology, Phenomenology, and the Sciences of Mind*, Cambridge, MA: Belknap Press.

———, and Stapleton, M. (2008), 'Making sense of sense-making: Reflections on enactive and extended mind theories', *Topoi*, 28: 1, pp. 23–30.

Tschacher, W. and Bergomi, C. (2011), 'Cognitive binding in schizophrenia: Weakened integration of temporal intersensory information', *Schizophrenia Bulletin*, 37: 1 2, pp. S13–S22.

Varela, F. (1977), 'The nervous system as a closed network', *Brain Theory Newsletter*, 2, pp. 66–67.

——— (1984), 'Two principles of self-organization', *Self-Organization and Management of Social Systems*, New York, NY: Springer Verlag, pp. 25–32.

——— (1996), 'Neurophenomenology: A methodological remedy for the hard problem', *Journal of Consciousness Studies*, 3: 4, pp. 330–49.

——— (1999), 'Present-time consciousness', *Journal of Consciousness Studies*, 6: 2–3, pp. 111–40.

———, Thompson, E. and Rosch, E. (1991), *The Embodied Mind: Cognitive Science and Human Experience*, Cambridge, MA: MIT Press.

Varela, F.J. (1991), 'Organism: A meshwork of selfless selves', in A.I. Tauber (ed.), *Organism and the Origins of Self*, New York, NY: Springer, pp. 79–107.

Van Manen, M. (2007), 'Phenomenology of practice', *Phenomenology and Practice*, 1: 1, pp. 11–30.

Van Orden, G. and Stephen, G., (2012), 'Is cognitive science a complexity science', *Topics in Cognitive Science*, 4, 1, pp. 3–6.

Vermersch, P. (2009), 'Describing the practice of introspection', in C. Petitmengin (ed.), *Ten Years of Viewing From Within: The Legacy of Francisco Varela*, Exeter, UK: Academic Press, pp. 20–57.

Warburton, E. (2011), 'Of meanings and movements: Re-languaging embodiment in dance phenomenology and cognition', *Dance Research Journal*, 43: 2, pp. 65–83.

Weber, A. and Varela, F. (2002), 'Life after Kant: Natural purposes and the autopoietic foundations of biological individuality', *Phenomenology and the Cognitive Sciences*, 1: 2, pp. 97–125.

Wilson, M. (2002), 'Six views of embodied cognition', *Psychonomic Bulletin & Review*, 9: 4, pp. 625–36.

Wilson, R. and Foglia, L. (2011), 'Embodied cognition', *Stanford Encyclopedia of Philosophy*. http://plato.stanford.edu/entries/embodied-cognition/. Accessed 15 January 2013.

Witowski, W. (2011), 'From Varela to a different phenomenology. Interview with Shaun Gallagher', *Avant*, 2: 2, pp. 77–84.

Notes

1   http://www.centrepompidou.fr/. Completed in 1977 as an initiative of former French President Pompidou, The Beaubourg continues to thrive as a multicultural center. André Malraux, the first minister of cultural affairs, gave rise to the idea. The Centre was designed by Italian architect Renzo Piano, British architect Richard Rogers and Italian architect Gianfranco Franchini, assisted by Ove Arup & Partners.

2   In this discussion of thinking in movement Sheets-Johnstone is describing improvisational dance. See M. Sheets-Johnstone (2011), *The Primacy of Movement* (2nd expanded edn, pp. 419–49; Chapter X in *The Corporeal Turn* (2009); and 'From movement to dance' (2012a).

3   For more than twenty years, Nancy Stark-Smith, pioneer of Contact Improvisation, has been interested in the brain-body interface as an act of bridging between dancemaking and language as a uniquely personal form of inquiry. This inquiry involves looking at the translation between dancing and writing and striving to develop a language for a movement experience while preserving its qualities. She writes: 'An inspiring dance can be quickly flattened when the mind closes in around it, trying…to define and enclose the experience (Stark-Smith 1982: 45). In one of her practices, she engages dancers in an experience that she has called 'hieroglyphs' (Stark-Smith 1982), a process part of which involves drawing quick, small 'glyphs' (pictograms) of the experiential process of moving. (See Appendix II for an example). Reflecting on these drawings – especially over a time of repeated practice – reveals a personal graphic language, evocative *data* for pondering brain processes underlying somatic states of attending to movement.

4   For reviews on the history of CS, see the opening chapter in Gallagher and Zahavi 2012: 1–14. For more specifics on the move toward embodiment theory, see Nagataki and Hirose 2007; Johnson 2008; and Shapiro 2010.

5   The concept of embodiment was debated among many academic disciplines, including philosophy, cognitive studies, neuroscience, ethnography, psychotherapy, the visual and performing arts, artificial intelligence, virtual reality and others (Bresler 2004). In addition, a number of other fields subscribed to embodied cognitive theory – for example, sociology, phenomenology; ecological psychology; neuroscience and neuropsychology; intelligence and robotics; and anthropology (Shapiro 2010).

6   Throughout the 1960s and 1970s, formalistic models of information processing gave way to models supporting ecological affordance and dynamical systems theory 'eco-systemic'

and 'enactive' models in which experience shaped cognition (Forte and Bonini 2010: 45). Futurist Gregory Bateson wrote that learning is unpredictable, dynamic, contextualized and emergent. Learning hinges on perceiving and interpreting differences between the self and the ecosystem (Bateson 1979). There is not one individual mind, but rather an interconnected web of mental processes (Bateson 1962).

7   Heidegger warns that phenomenology 'never makes things easier, but only more difficult' (2000: 12). He agrees with those who feel that phenomenology lacks effectiveness or utility if one hopes to do something practically useful with it: ' "Nothing comes" of philosophy; "you can't do anything with it." These two turns of phrase, which are especially current among teachers and researchers in the sciences, express observations that have their indisputable correctness…[It] consists in the prejudice that one can evaluate philosophy according to everyday standards that one would otherwise employ to judge the utility of bicycles or the effectiveness of mineral baths' (2000: 13). The practicality of a phenomenology of practice should not be sought in instrumental action, efficiency or technical efficacy. And yet, that does not mean that phenomenology cannot have practical value.

Chapter 3

Researching Dance Cognition – Task-Based Analysis

Every language is clumsy and inadequate when it comes to dynamics.

(Maxine Sheets-Johnstone 2009: 363)

Overview

How can researchers capture the complexity of cognitive processes in dancemaking? One possible model is 'task-based analysis' from human movement science.[1,2] *Tasks* readily promote efficiency because they contain features called *constraints*. Constraints shape temporal, spatial and effort dynamics within movement patterns, enabling ease of task execution. Constraints consist of the combined characteristics of the person doing the task, and the context and demands of the task. The constraints involved in making a cup of coffee in your kitchen, for example, automatically organize the task. That is, your familiarity with the location and shape of the coffee mug help shape the dynamics of reaching and grasping. Improvising with ten other dancers on a mountainous terrain calls upon a whole other set of constraints. This chapter describes the rudiments of task-based analysis apropos to dance research. We first suggest operationalizing the term *dancemaking* to increase scientific rigor. Second, we provide an overview of task-based analysis from the perspective of human movement science. Finally, we provide several current examples of task-based approaches to studying embodied cognition in dancemaking.

Focusing in…

- What definition(s) capture the scope of dancemaking?
- Why is it important to differentiate dancemaking from other forms of skilled movement?
- What is a task? What is a constraint? Provide examples of your own personal (psychophysical) constraints that have impacted on learning structured dance phrases (either facilitating your ability to accomplish the phrase or challenging your ability).
- How can task-based analysis provide a model for the indirect study of embodied cognitive processes in dance?
- Dancers: describe how you *marked* a recently learned phrase or section of choreography you learned. Non-dancers: describe how you used your hands or other body parts to *code* and remember key information.

Experiential prelude

For dance novices and aficionados

Reflect on your day. Take a moment to jot down five tasks you accomplished since you got up this morning, no matter how pedestrian or seemingly insignificant. Reflect on your movement patterns in completing several of these common, everyday tasks. How did these *choreographies* play out? What were the motivating factors for getting them done? Did you vary from your habitual ways of completing any one of them? Which tasks were the most taxing – mentally and physically? How did you lower the amount of effort to get things done? What impact did varying the task have? Did you find yourself improvising to accomplish any task? Do the exercise again sometime, deliberately trying out new means of accomplishment.

For dancers

Can you compare your strategies for completing tasks in dance with strategies in everyday life? List tasks assigned in a recent dance experience. Was this event structured or improvisational? Who asked you to complete these tasks – teacher or choreographer? List all the elements that constrained your focus of attention – psychophysical, affective, environmental etc. How did the constraints help or hinder in organizing and completing the task? Compare a more structured dance context with improvising on your own. In what ways does the structured dance context tax you mentally/physically? What tools (psychophysical strategies) did you use to cope with task demands? What constraints did you employ while improvising? How did the two experiences differ?

Introduction

Researching dance cognition utilizes two main methodologies – direct and indirect. Direct analysis requires technology – imaging scanners and other methods that capture neural activity *online*. Indirect methods include movement observation and analysis. At this point in time, direct methods lack *eco-validity*. The current state of the art of most neuro-technologies limit recording brain processes during full-out dancing. Neuro-imaging can record the brain's implicit processes while watching dance (Calvo-Merino et al. 2005) or imagining dance (Hökelmann and Blaser 2009), for example, but not actually dancing. The ability to capture the full-blown dynamics of dance performance awaits further technological advancement.

Task-based analysis offers an indirect approach to studying dance cognition. Many tasks are embedded in virtually every dance context – instructed or improvisational. How do the personal characteristics of the dancer(s), the demands of the task and the environmental context shape the movement outcome? What then can be inferred from task accomplishment about cognition? In order to begin to understand task-based dance research – or any dance research for that matter – it is first important to define 'dance'. Below we've described a few ways to think constructively about operationalizing the term.

What is dance(making)?

Whether celebrating physical virtuosity or not (Hanna 2001), dance is a form of artistic communication that *becomes* itself through experimentation *of* itself (Stevens et al. 2003; Vaughan 1990; Hanna 1979; author's italics). At the same time, what and how dance communicates may not be explicit. Dance is not necessarily *about* anything. It does not necessarily describe or explain concepts.[3] Dance performance 'ex-scribes' rather than describes (Stern 2011: 237). 'The body's ambiguity – its peculiar complexity...refuses either naturalistic or intellectualistic descriptions...[and] does not explain anything...but rather begs further explanation' (Adamson 2005: 186). The goals of a dance may, in fact, be more *implicit*, aimed at emancipating the body, movement, thought or ideology (Kozel 2005).

Meaning emerges from the complex confluence of many internal dynamics (kinetic, kinematic, kinesthetic, somatic, empathic and affective). External dynamics are important, too (spatial, melodic, architectural or other features of the environment). It is in this multisensory, multimodal immersion in movement that new movement forms emerge and take on meaning (Legrand and Ravn 2009; deLahunta, Barnard and McGregor 2009). Dance transforms a material body into a dynamical one, thereby extending its communicative capacities. The 'is-ness' of dance (both what it knows and how it knows) is fueled by the moment-by-moment changes in movement dynamics. These embody kinetic and affective power that becomes palpably sensed and meaningful. The possibilities for new dance forms are limitless, and the emergence and transfer of meaning can be tangible, intangible or even non-tangible, depending on context (Thelen 1995; Howe, Davidson and Sloboda 1998).

At the same time, other movement styles and forms also exhibit powerful dynamics, regardless of whether the movement is functional or dysfunctional or the mover able-bodied or otherwise-abled. Athletes, and other experts of psychophysical practices such as martial arts, dramatic arts, mime, circus arts and other performative arts, also exhibit powerful dynamics – capabilities that extend as well to virtual- or robotic movement (Yarrow, Brown and Krakauer 2009). What definition, then, captures the particularities and scope of dance? The boundaries–whether artistic, functional or other–have stretched so far, that the questions as to what dance *is* or what dance is *about*, lose their relevance (Owen Clark 2011).[4]

At its most abstract, a dancer has been described as a 'stabilized self-destabilizing system, open to internal transformation' (Melrose 2009: 25). Through this lens, subjective associations with music and storytelling, sociocultural ethnicity and personal expressiveness are minimized. Also avoided are mechanistic terms such as the dancing body as an 'instrument' (Balanchine n.d.), a 'vehicle' (Hawkins 1991) or a 'mechanism' (Beavers 2008). From the phenomenological perspective, the dancing body is not a material thing separate from dance, but a holistic gestalt manifesting as dance. The body-in-dance is a process of being in the world – 'besouled, bespirited and beminded…[and]… inseparable' (Fraleigh 1987: 11, 31).

But dance is more than phenomenal. Dance is research that contains many complex tangible and non-tangible phenomena. It is a continually shifting movement fabric in which many elements intrinsic to dancer and context converge to become *the dance*. Dancers dance 'to formulate, explain or unravel and communicate complex ideas' (Flink and Odde 2012; Glass and Stevens 2005; Hagendoorn 2002). In this respect, dance exhibits *dynamical complexity*.[5] These complex phenomena are not readily measurable and may even be resistant to reductionist analysis (Newell 2008; Bläsing et al. 2012). The gestalt emerges without an overarching executive mental agent, plan or program proposed from the outset.

Further, 'the' dance is not a unidimensional, undifferentiated act or event (Lepecki 2004). Dancemaking engages many nested spheres of activity, enfolded and enmeshed. Dance movements are 'continuous and discontinuous' (King 2003: 16), 'sequential but not necessarily segmented or detachable…spilling over' from one movement to the next (Sheets-Johnstone 2009: 34), proceeding 'forwards, then backwards, and then forwards again…reflexively' (Hanstein 1999: 29). Space-time-effort phenomena function paradoxically within dance as continuous and discrete events (Jones 2009). Each event becomes a node of interest within the fractal whole (Massumi 2003). The time line of events also is marked by interruptions, planned (May et al. 2011) and unplanned. These interruptions may themselves serve as self-organizing strategies that take the dance to another level (Protopapa 2011). With the intent to communicate aesthetically, dancers exert a 'tension' [in the task of] retaining a kind of fidelity' to the dancemaking process (Protopapa 2011: 104).

Finally, 'the' dance is an illustration of embodied cognitive complexity. Dancemaking is an inquiry of the body and mind in motion – an ongoing negotiation of who, what, which, when, why, where and how within time and space.[6] How, then, do researchers investigate complex mental phenomena of dancemaking? One way is to consider dancemaking *tasks* and their impact. The *task-based approach* affords researchers an inroad into investigating complex mental phenomena.

Tasks and constraints

On a day-to-day basis, we attend to many tasks – getting dressed, working at a computer, driving a car or weaving in and out of foot traffic while walking to work. Tasks organize us. They define the nature and focus of our attention. They control our movement patterns. How can tasks do this?

Tasks organize activities by simplifying goal accomplishment. Tasks contain embedded features called 'constraints'.[7] They at once afford opportunities for organizing movement and at the same time limit relationships (Smith 2006; Kelso 1995). They provide a coherent framework for understanding how coordination patterns emerge in goal directed activity (Glazier and Davids 2009: 32). Unlike robots whose movement constraints are 'hardwired', human beings are living, adaptive systems. Coordination unfolds temporally, spatially and dynamically out of a confluence of flexible constraints. Human constraints then, are 'softly assembled' (Thelen and Smith 1996: 122). They enable flexible relationships and outcomes. Even our reflexes are not permanently fixed or obligatory. Take walking, for example. A dancer walks differently depending on whether the walk is in a familiar neighborhood, a postmodern dance walk or a ballet walk – or, when wearing high heels (Schaefer and Lindenberger 2013) versus bare feet or ballet slippers. To 'walk like a dancer' influences coordination differently than pedestrian walking.

Three interacting task constraints impact on cognition within dancemaking: (1) the psychophysical characteristics of the individual dancer, group of dancers and the audience; (2) the movement method and selections (evolving phrase material); and (3) the environmental context. These features interact to coordinate unique movement patterns. Constraints might include the dancer's anthropomorphic- and other bio-characteristics (leg length, level of fitness, etc.), the choreographer's intentions, the performance space and the weather. While western contemporary dance cannot be reduced to one style or genre, commonly accepted movement patterns and vocabulary act as constraints in helping dancers develop embodied knowledge. These act as specific codes for spatial, temporal and aesthetic requirements (Parvianien 2002). For example, Rudolph Laban's conceptions of time, weight, direction and flow (Laban 1971) provide a common vocabulary of constraints that shape movement performance.

Task constraints, then, act as a kind of *organizational logic*. Constraints are so embedded in everyday life tasks that we rarely think about their unique organizational facility for bringing about *efficiency* and *effectiveness*.[8] At the same time, tasks require a good deal of cognitive processing (the work of thinking). For example, tasks impose a 'load' or burden on working memory. This term, 'cognitive load', comes from cognitive psychology, and describes the brain's capability to handle the finite amount of working memory (Paas, Renkel and Sweller 2004; Kahnemann 1973).[9] It is commonly understood that the capacity for human memory is roughly 5–9 bits of information at once (thus, the seven-digit phone number) (Miller 1956). Despite this, humans rarely are aware of the mental effort that tasks elicit (Vilar et al. 2012). Many tasks operate unconsciously and automatically. Further, there are many ways to 'off-load' cognitive work onto the environment (Wilson 2002: 626), thereby reducing cognitive load. Programming important numbers on your cell phone is one example of off-loading tasks. The memory on your smartphone frees up your own memory from the burden of remembering multiple phone numbers.

Finally, constraints act as 'control parameters' (Newell 1986: 343). They set limits on ways to move. Without constraints, every time humans were faced with the same task, they would be confronted by a potentially infinite number of ways for accomplishment. Constraints, therefore, simplify complexity and make life easier. At the same time, constraint does not mean restraint. Paradoxically, the limits imposed by the constraints afford a means of developing (rather than dissipating) the developing dance. They facilitate coordination by at once reducing redundancy and at the same time, providing inroads for expanding and developing movement material. They operate 'iteratively',[10] allowing re-entry into the task for further thematic explication. Reducing redundancy and variability fine-tunes these patterns of coordination (Patterson 2001). Whether the dance is improvisational or more instructed, task constraints deepen relationships (Sgorbati 2005; Sgorbati, Climer and Haas 2013). As movement dynamics are explored and taxed, the context changes and deepens developmentally. Changing any one constraint within a phrase – the spatial relations, timing, rhythms etc. – opens possibilities for creating new movement and expression.

Embodied cognition: three examples of task-based research

Tasks rein in parameters so that key aspects of the dance context can be repeatedly located and analyzed. Because of this, task-based analysis provides a model not only for investigating movement patterns and relationships, but also for indirectly examining cognitive processes within dancemaking. The following studies represent three examples of approaches to studying cognitive processes through task-based/constraints-led analysis.[11]

In the physical tasks of dancemaking, dancers generate problems as well as solve them. Every phase and phrase of dancing calls upon different cognitive strategies (learning structured movement, improvising, marking, rehearsing in the studio, rehearsing in the theater and performing). Many phases of work organize the dancer and the dance from its conception to its final performance (assuming here a studio-to-theater-based professional dance experience). Examples include (but are not limited to) the pre-preparation phase, the learning phase, the formally setting phrase (Jola 2010), marking (Kirsh 2011; Warburton 2013) and the rehearsing, performing and revising stages (Jola, Ehrenberg and Reynolds 2012). Different processes and skills are needed within each stage/phase. Verbal codes and rhythmic or movement chunking and marking, for example, serve as shorthand ways of coding complex information. These codes reduce the cognitive burden subject to the volume of information (see below for examples). These codes serve multiple purposes: to assist memory, reduce mental effort and generally help keep dancers on task.

1. Imagery prompts as constraints on new movement creation

Imagining action is a powerful act of embodied cognition (Kosslyn, Thompson and Ganis 2006). An image acts as a 'cognitive' constraint by influencing space-, time and effort-shape dynamics. Dance choreographers and teachers often provide their dancers with imagery as improvisational prompts to stimulate new movement creation. These prompts become the dancers' tasks in developing new movement material. Using images as prompts for movement creation provides ample ways of studying focus of attention, organization and decision-making. Imagery generates action. First, an image can arise intuitively, simply from exploring movement; second, images can shape and alter the dynamics of an ongoing movement; and third, images can allow the dancer to project outside of self, offering ways to observe the self in interacting with space, time and others.

For more than a decade, British choreographer Wayne McGregor has been collaborating with scientists to explore the effects of imagery on movement creation.[12] May and colleagues (May et al. 2011) focused on McGregor's problem-solving approach to creating movement through visual imagery. McGregor chose highly 'spatial-praxic' visual imagery. Here, dancers visualized objects or volumes outside the body to manipulate or interact with, as well as imagining images colored by emotional tone of a narrative. His instructions clarified task intent and stimulated decision-making processes. Researchers could observe and document behavior via multiple qualitative questionnaires and fMRI recordings. Results were surprising and counterintuitive. By reflecting on (and categorizing) their experiences, dancers gained new insights into their mental habits of improvising with imagery prompts. The dancers were surprised to learn the realities of their perceptual focus. While they believed they were focusing on physical/bodily aspects in creating movement, results showed that they were, in fact, focusing more on the conceptual aspects. Further, choreographer McGregor also gained insight into ways to 'communicate more productively [to his dancers] about the properties of the task-based instructions' (May et al. 2011: 405). Results offered inroads into mutual processes of observation, reflection and articulation that stimulated new inquiry.

2. Environment as constraint on improvisation

Torrents and colleagues (2010) analyzed the responses and movement characteristics of Contact Improvisation dancers in a constrained setting. Here, the catalyst for movement generation was not imagery per se, but the dynamics emerging from two major constraints: a tight performance setting and the instructional demands made on dancers. Four experienced contact improvisers performed duets in a constrained 10 × 10 meter space. Demands were made on each dancer to couple with one of the other three dancers in specific ways and intervals. The resulting contact duets created a new 'system for movement' analysis (Torrents 2010: 2). Three outside dance experts analyzed video recordings using the Observational System of Motor Skills (OSMOS) (Castañer et al. 2008; Castañer and Camerino 2006). This interactive video coding program captures movements such as axial stability skills, level changing stability skills, locomotor skills and manipulative skills when dancing – not only as events, but also as temporal patterns (frequency of occurrence), as they combine and/or change. Dancers wrote down their reflections. The researchers were able to define and describe a number of events within the improvisational context.

3. Marking as constraint on working memory

Marking is encapsulating key aspects of a movement phrase by using one part of the body (e.g., hands) or the whole body. Marking is a kind of *sketch* of the complete movement phrase. In marking, dancers don't dance full out, but rather rehearse steps in a shorthand manner. This 'attenuated' or 'reduced' version (Warburton et al. 2013: 1) of the choreographed phrase acts as a 'representation vehicle' (Kirsh 2010: 2864). This shorthand version is abstracted from the real time-space-efforts of the fully performed movement. Marking compresses the space, timing and energy level of execution of the movement phrase, replacing full-out movements with much smaller gestures of the lower limbs or hands (Warburton et al. 2013). The resulting movement is smaller in spatial representation and easier in terms of effort. At the same time, these small gestures represent the whole context, helping dancers to perceive and remember the conceptual whole.

The main purpose traditionally has been to save physical energy (Homans 2010). Marking allows dancers to capture key space-time-effort qualities within the phrase and augment them within memory through repetition and reinforcement without energy expenditure. More recently, however, marking has been viewed as a means of assisting memory (Kirsh 2010) and improving the efficiency of motor learning (Warburton 2013). Marking reduces both the physical and 'cognitive load' or burden of thinking (Cowen 2000; Paas, Renkel and Sweller 2004). In dance, this 'load' results from the act of learning, performing and remembering complex movement material.

What is evocative from the cognitive standpoint is how marking acts as a 'complementary strategy' to 'reduce cognitive overload' (Kirsh 1995: 1). In daily living, humans need to reduce the burden on working memory in coping with the complexity of our actions. We use our bodies to condense and parse information processing, constructing mini-gestures to remember names, numbers and events. The body becomes a landscape for devising creative strategies. These strategies at once ease the load on cognition as well as 'enhance our cognitive performance' (Kirsh 1995). By such strategies, we reduce the time and effort needed to actually execute a task, thereby still 'learning' and 'remembering' but with more ease. 'Such complementary strategies are mental "trade-offs" – speed-accuracy, speed-problem size, speed-robustness' (Kirsh 1995: 214).

Marking hones perception and attention to key details of the movement as well as sharpens memory (Kirsh 1995; Warburton et al. 2013). It is a cognitive strategy where dancers can 'harness their bodies to drive thought deeper than through mental simulation and unaided thinking alone' (Kirsh 2011). Although considered similar to covert mental practice of motor imagery (mental rehearsal), neurologically, it is a different task with different goals. Marking incorporates real time-space values. Effort values are approximated and minimized, but usually more than those primed in mental rehearsal. Last, marking helps dancers understand more of the choreographer/teacher's intentions. They are practicing, as it were, 'the empathic imperative in dancing' (Warburton 2011: 76).

Further, marking is not one undifferentiated event. Different needs, intentions and goals shape both its uses and outcomes. At the University of California, San Diego, cognitive scientist David Kirsh studied the structure and function of marking, using a systematic video coding system called ELAN, which coded the formal vocabulary established by the research team as well as participating dancers' interviews. These marking methods appear to be very individualized, internal and personal, even with the external appearance of similarity. How each dancer interprets the flow of the weight of the body through space and time has its nuances. Kirsh and his colleagues uncovered three functional uses of marking: 'Marking-for-self', 'marking–for-others' and 'joint-marking'. With each functional category dancers used their bodies to sketch out the relevant variables of a phrase for themselves, for the larger performance space events and for tight coupling in a duet, respectively (Kirsh 2010: 2865).

Kirsh asked the question: 'Is it plausible to see marking as a vehicle of thought?' Kirsh sees the complexity of marking as first a 'type of gestural semiotic system, possibly like a linguistic code'. Second, marking 'primes' the neuromuscular system. Third, marking augments our experience and its agency by 'projecting' onto external targets (Kirsh 2010: 2866, 2867). In a different way, Edward (Ted) Warburton views marking as providing 'a scaffold to mentally project more detailed structure onto the architecture *and* poetry of the dance…[putting] cognitive and psychomotor processes in the service of empathic response and ultimately movement expression' (Warburton 2013: 76).

In 2012, Warburton and colleagues designed a study to test the cognitive effects of marking on learning complex dance phrases. The researchers hypothesized that high-level dance was not only physically, but also cognitively demanding (ibid.: 2). They predicted that marking would confer cognitive benefits that would result in better movement performance. The method consisted of recruiting thirty-eight advanced ballet dancers who were divided into two groups – the marking group and the repetitive practice group. Two complex routines were learned and rehearsed: one group spending part of rehearsal time marking the phrases, the other group rehearsing full out each time. As predicted, the marking group performed better on the final test phrases than the group who rehearsed full out.

While it may seem intuitive that rehearsing dance phrases full out would benefit performance, results from this study suggest otherwise. It appears a better strategy to save the brain 'from mentally allocating resources in attending to all aspects of performance' (Warburton et al. 2013: 2). Full-out physical exertion can impose an excessive cognitive burden or load. Too many resources are allocated in controlling body mechanics, balance and other factors, rather than being able to attend to the actual movement material at hand. Marking reduces this cognitive burden, helping elite dancers program the movement while saving cognitive resources that may be more readily depleted in physical performance. Marking and other strategies 'may allow dancers to physically rehearse some aspects of the performance (e.g., timing, head and arm movements, or movement qualities) and mentally rehearse other aspects (e.g., the choreographic sequence, with the turn represented in the appropriate place in the sequence) while eliminating altogether the need to allocate attention to still other aspects (e.g., maintaining balance during a turn or reorienting oneself in space after a turn)' (Warburton 2013: 2).

Summary

Taken together, these studies address many elements of embodied cognition: perception, attention, intention, judgment and decision-making. The task-based model provides a framework that goes beyond analyzing movement towards understanding cognitive- and other processes that afford the various outcomes. In summary, the model affords researchers ways of investigating complex cognitive processes that might ordinarily remain elusive or resistant to analysis.

Explorations are located in Appendix II.

References

Adamson, T. (2005), 'Measure for measure: The reliance of human knowledge on things of the world', *Ethics and the Environment*, 10: 2, pp. 175–94.

Balanchine, G. (n.d.), Attributed to George Balanchine (n.d.), http://www.goodreads.com/quotes/332275-dancers-are-instruments-like-a-piano-the-choreographer-plays. Accessed 18 August 2013.

Beavers, W. (2008), 'Locating technique', in M. Bales and R. Nettl-Fiol (eds.), *The Body Eclectic: Evolving Practices in Dance Training*, Chicago, IL: University of Illinois Press, pp. 126–33.

Bläsing, B., Calvo-Merino, B., Cross, E.S., Jola, C., Honisch, J. and Stevens, C.J. (2012), 'Neurocognitive control in dance perception and performance', *Acta Psychologica*, 139, pp. 300–08.

Brown, S., Martinez, M.J. and Parsons, L.M. (2006), 'The neural basis of human dance', *Cerebral Cortex*, 16: 8, pp. 1157–67.

Calvo-Merino, B., Glaser, D.E., Grèzes, J., Passingham, R.E. and Haggard, P. (2005), 'Action observation and acquired motor skills: An fMRI study with expert dancers', *Cerebral Cortex*, 15: 8, pp. 1243–49.

Castaner, M. and Camerino, O. (2006), 'Manifestaciones basicas de la motricidad', Lleida: INEFC-UdL.

Castaner, M., Torrents, C., Anguera, M.T. and Dinosova, M. (2008), 'Identifying and analysing motor skills answers in the corporal expression and dance through OSMOS', in A.J. Spink, M.R. Ballintijn, N. Bogers et al. (eds.), *Proceedings of 6th International Conference on Methods and Techniques in Behavioral Research*, Maastricht, the Netherlands: Noldus Information Technology, pp. 158–60.

Chow, J.Y., Davids, K., Button, C., Shuttleworth, R., Renshaw, I. and Araújo, D. (2006), 'Nonlinear pedagogy: A constraints-led framework for understanding emergence of game play and movement skills', *Nonlinear Dynamics, Psychology, and Life Sciences*, 10: 1, pp. 71–103.

Chow, J.Y., Davids, K., Button, C., Shuttleworth, R., Renshaw, I. and Araújo, D. (2007), 'The role of nonlinear pedagogy in physical education', *Review of Educational Research*, 77: 3, pp. 251–78.

Cowan, N. (2000), 'The magical number 4 in short-term memory: A reconsideration of mental storage capacity', *Behavioral and Brain Sciences*, 24: 1, pp. 87–185.

Covello, V.T. (2003), *Keeping Your Head in a Crisis: Responding to Communication Challenges Posed by Bioterrorism and Emerging Infectious Diseases*, Association of State and Territorial Health Officers (ASTHO).

Davids, K., Button, C. and Bennett, S. (2008), *Dynamics of Skill Acquisition: A Constraints-Led Approach*, Champaign, IL: Human Kinetics.

Davids, K., Button, C. and Newell, K.M. (2006), *Movement System Variability*, Champaign, IL: Human Kinetics.

deLahunta, S., Barnard, P. and McGregor, W. (2009), 'Augmenting choreography: Using insights and inspiration from science' in J. Butterworth and L. Wildschut (eds.), *Contemporary Choreography: A Critical Reader*, New York, NY: Routledge, pp. 431–48.

Finke, R.A., Ward, T.B. and Smith, S.M. (1996), *Creative Cognition: Theory, Research, and Applications*, Cambridge: MA: MIT Press.

Flink, C. and Odde, D. (2012), 'Science + dance = bodystorming', *Cellular Biology*, 22, pp. 613–16.

Fraleigh, S.N. (1987), *Dance and the Lived Body: A Descriptive Aesthetics*, Pittsburgh, PA: University of Pittsburgh Press.

Gallagher, S. (2006), *How the Body Shapes the Mind*, New York, NY: Oxford University Press.

Gallese, V. (2009), 'Mirror neurons, embodied simulation, and the neural basis of social identification', *Psychoanalytic Dialogues*, 19, pp. 519–36.

Glass, R. and Stevens, C. (2005), 'Choreographic cognition: Investigating the psychological processes involved in contemporary dance' in K. Vincs (ed.), *Dance Rebooted: Initializing the Grid*, Conference Proceedings, Ausdance National, December 2004, http://ausdance.org.au/articles/details/choreographic-cognition. Accessed 8 February 2013.

Glazier, P.S. and Davids, K. (2009), 'Constraints on the complete optimization of human motion', *Sports Medicine*, 39: 1, pp. 15–28.

Hagendoorn, I.G. (2002), 'Emergent patterns in dance improvisation and choreography', Proceedings of the International Conference on Complex Systems. Online: http://www.ivarhagendoorn.com/research/emergent-patterns-in-dance-improvisation-and-choreography. Accessed 30 November 2012.

Hanna, J.L. (1979), *To Dance Is Human: A Theory of Non-Verbal Communication*, Chicago: University of Chicago Press.

Hanna, J.L. (2001), 'The language of dance', *Journal of Physical Education, Recreation and Dance*, 72, 4, pp. 40–45.

Hanstein, P. (1999), 'From idea to research proposal: Balancing the systematic and serendipitous' in S.N. Fraleigh and P. Hanstein (eds.), *Researching Dance: Evolving Modes of Inquiry*, Pittsburgh, PA: University of Pittsburgh Press, pp. 22–61.

Hawkins, A.M., (1991), *Moving From Within: A New Method for Dance Making*, Atlanta, GA: Cappella Books.

Hökelmann, A. and Blaser, P. (2009), 'Mental reproduction of a dance choreography and its effects on physiological fatigue in dancers', *Journal of Human Sport and Exercise*, 4: 2, pp. 129–41.

Homans, J. (2010), *Apollo's Angels: A History of Ballet*, New York, NY: Random House.

Howe, J.J.A., Davidson, J.W. and Sloboda, J.A. (1998), 'Innate talents: Reality or myth', *Behavioural and Brain Sciences*, 21, pp. 399–442.

Jola, C. (2010), 'Research and choreography: Merging dance and cognitive neuroscience' in B. Bläsing, M. Puttke and T. Schack (eds.), *The Neurocognition of Dance: Mind, Movement and Motor Skills*, London: Routledge, pp. 203–34.

Jola, C., Ehrenberg, S. and Reynolds, D. (2012), 'The experience of watching dance: Phenomenological-neuroscience duets', *Phenomenology and the Cognitive Sciences*, 11: 1, pp. 17–37.

Jones, S. (2009), 'At the still point: T.S. Eliot, dance and modernism', *Dance Research Journal*, 41: 2, pp. 31–51.

Kahneman, D. (1973), *Attention and Effort,* Englewood Cliffs, NJ: Prentice-Hall.

Kelso, J. (1995), *Dynamic Patterns: the Self-Organization of Brain and Behavior,* Cambridge, MA: MIT Press.

King, K. (2003), *Writing in Motion: Body-Language-Technology*, Middletown, CT: Wesleyan University Press.

Kirsh, D. (1995), 'Complementary strategies: Why we use our hands when we think' in J.D. Moore and J.F. Lehman (eds.), *Proceedings of the Seventeenth Annual Conference of the Cognitive Science Society*, pp. 212–17. http://adrenaline.ucsd.edu/kirsh/articles/cogsci95/cogsci95.htm. Accessed 13 February 2013.

Kirsh, D. (2010), *Thinking With the Body*, in S. Ohlsson and R. Catrambone (eds.), *Proceedings of the 32nd Annual Conference of the Cognitive Science Society*, Austin, TX: Cognitive Science Society, pp. 2864–69.

Kirsh, D. (2011), 'Creative cognition in choreography' in *Proceedings of 2nd International Conference on Computational Creativity*, Mexico City, Mexico, http://adrenaline.ucsd.edu/Kirsh/publications.html. Accessed 14 February 2013.

Kirsh, D. et al. (2009), 'Choreographic methods for creating novel, high quality dance', *5th International Workshop on Design and Semantics of Form and Movement*, http://adrenaline.ucsd.edu/Kirsh/publications.html. Accessed 14 February 2013.

Kugler, P.N., Kelso, J.A.S. and Turvey, M.T. (1982), 'On the control and coordination of naturally developing systems' in J.A.S. Kelso and J.E. Clark (eds.), *The Development of Movement Control and Co-ordination*, New York, NY: Wiley, pp. 5–78.

Kozel, S. (2005). 'Connective tissue: the flesh of the network' in K. Vincs (ed.), *Dance Rebooted: Initializing the Grid*, Conference Proceedings, Ausdance National, December 2004. http://ausdance.org.au/articles/details/connective-tissue-the-flesh-of-the-network. Accessed 28 April 2012.

Kosslyn, S.M., Thompson, W.L. and Ganis, G. (2006), *The Case for Mental Imagery*, Cambridge, MA: Harvard University Press.

Laban, R. (1971), *The Mastery of Movement*, 3rd edn, London: MacDonald and Evans.

Legrand, D. and Ravn, S. (2009), 'Perceiving subjectivity in bodily movement: The case of dancers', *Phenomenology and the Cognitive Science*s, 8: 3, pp. 389–408.

Lepecki, A. (2004), *Of the Presence of the Body: Essays on Dance and Performance Theory*, Middletown, CT: Wesleyan University Press.

Massumi, B. (2003), 'The archive of experience' in J. Brouwer and A. Mulder (eds.), *Information Is Alive: Art and Theory on Archiving and Retrieving Data*, Rotterdam, NL: V2 Organisatie/EU European Culture 2000 Program, 2003, pp. 142–51. http://www.brianmassumi.com/textes/Archive%20of%20Experience.pdf. Accessed 11 February 2013.

May, J., Calvo-Merino, B., deLahunta, S., McGregor, W, Cusack, R., Owen, A. and Barnard, P. (2011), 'Points in mental space: An interdisciplinary study of imagery in movement creation', *Dance Research*, 29: 2, pp. 402–30.

Melrose, S. (2009), 'Expert-intuitive processing and the logics of production: Struggles in (the wording of) creative decision-making in "dance" ', in J. Butterworth and L. Wildschut (eds.), *Contemporary Choreography: A Critical Reader*, New York, NY: Routledge, pp. 23–44.

Miller, G.A. (1956), 'The magical number seven, plus or minus two: Some limits on our capacity for processing information', *Psychology Review*, 63, pp. 81–97.

Nagrin, D. (1999), *The Six Questions: Acting Technique for Dance*, Pittsburgh, PA: University of Pittsburgh Press.

Newell, C. (2008). 'The class as a learning entity (complex adaptive system): An idea from complexity science and educational research', *SFU Educational Review*, 2: 1, pp. 5–17.

Newell, K.M. (1986), 'Constraints on the development of coordination', *Motor Development in Children: Aspects of Coordination and Control*, 34, pp. 341–60.

Nielsen, J.B. and Cohen, L.G. (2008), 'The Olympic brain. Does corticospinal plasticity play a role in acquisition of skills required for high-performance sports?', *Journal of Physiology*, 586, pp. 65–70.

Owen Clark, J. (2011), 'Dance and subtraction: Notes on Alain Badiou's Inaesthetics', *Dance Research Journal*, 43: 2, pp. 50–64.

Paas, F., Renkel, A. and Sweller, J. (2004), 'Cognitive load theory: Instructional implications of the interaction between information structures and cognitive architecture', *Instructional Science*, 32, pp. 1–8.

Patterson, T.S. (2001), 'Constraints: An integrated viewpoint', *Illuminaire*, 7: 1, pp. 30–37.

Parviainen, J. (2002), 'Epistemology reflections on dance', *Dance Research Journal*, 34: 1, pp. 11–18.

Protopapa, E. (2011), 'Performance-making as interruption in practice-led research', *Choreographic Practices*, 2: 1, pp. 103–11.

Renshaw, I., Davids, K. and Savelsbergh, G.J.P. (2012), *Motor Learning in Practice: A Constraints-Led Approach*, New York, NY: Taylor and Francis (Routledge).

Renshaw, I., Chow, J.Y., Davids, K. and Hammond, J. (2010), 'A constraints-led perspective to understanding skill acquisition and game play: A basis for integration of motor learning theory and physical education praxis?', *Physical Education and Sport Pedagogy*, 15: 2, pp. 117–37.

Reynolds, D. and Reason, M. (2012), *Kinesthetic Empathy in Creative and Cultural Practices*, Bristol/Chicago: Intellect Books.

Schaefer, S. and Lindenberger, U. (2013), 'Thinking while walking: Experienced high-heel walkers flexibly adjust their gait', *Frontiers in Psychology*, 4, pp. 316–25.

Sgorbati, S. (2005). Emergent improvisation. http://emergentimprovisation.org/essay.html. Accessed 20 December 2012.

Sgorbati, S., Climer, E. and Haas, M.L. (2013), *Emergent Improvisation*, Chapbook 4, *Contact Quarterly*, 38: 2, pp. 1–57.

Sheets-Johnstone, M. (2009), *The Corporeal Turn: An Interdisciplinary Reader*, Charlottesville, VA: Imprint Academic.

Serrien, D.J., Ivry, R.B. and Swinnen, S.P. (2007), 'The missing link between action and cognition', *Progress in Neurobiology*, 82: 2, pp. 95–107.

Smith, L.B. (2006), 'Movement matters: The contributions of Esther Thelen', *Biological Theory*, 1: 1, pp. 87–89.

Stern, N. (2011), 'The Implicit Body as Performance: Analyzing Interactive Art', *Leonardo*, 44: 3, pp. 233–38.

Stevens, C., Malloch, S., McKechnie, S. and Steven, N. (2003), 'Choreographic cognition: The time-course and phenomenology of creating a dance', *Pragmatics & Cognition*, 11: 2, pp. 297–326.

Thelen, E. (1995), 'Motor development: A new synthesis', *American Psychologist*, 50: 2, pp. 79–95.

Thelen, E. and Smith, L.B. (1994), *A Dynamics Systems Approach to the Development of Cognition and Action*, Cambridge, MA: Bradford Books/MIT Press.

Torrents, C., Castanea, M., Dinusova, M. and Anguera, M.T. (2010), 'Discovering new ways of moving: Observational analysis of motor creativity while dancing Contact Improvisation and the influence of a partner', *Journal of Creative Behavior*, http://www.fmh.utl.pt/spertlab/images/files/TorrentsEtAl2010_Observational_analysis_in_dance.pdf. Accessed 12 February 2013.

Vaughan, D. (1990), Merce Cunningham in S. Sontag and R. Francis, *Cage, Cunningham, Johns: Dancers on a Plane in Memory of Their Feeling*, London: Thames and Hudson, pp. 81–87.

Vilar, L., Araujo, D., Davids, K. and Button, C. (2012), 'The role of ecological dynamics in analyzing performance in team sports', *Sports Medicine*, 42: 1, pp. 1–10.

Warburton, E.C. (2011), 'Of meanings and movements: Re-languaging embodiment in dance phenomenology and cognition', *Dance Research Journal*, 43: 2, pp. 65–84.

Warburton, E.C., Wilson, M., Lynch, M. and Cuykendall, S. (2013), 'The cognitive benefits of movement reduction: Evidence from dance marking', *Psychological Science*, 24: 9, pp. 1732–39.

Wilson, M. (2002), 'Six views of embodied cognition', *Psychonomic Bulletin and Review*, 9, pp. 625–636.

Yarrow, K., Brown, P. and Krakauer, J.W. (2009), 'Inside the brain of an elite athlete: The neural processes that support high achievement in sports', *Nature Reviews Neuroscience*, 10, pp. 585–96.

Notes

1 Cognitive psychology divides researching mental processes into two broad categories: implicit and explicit. Task-based research can be categorized more readily as explicit. The chapter omits an enormous body of 'implicit' research in dance (Warburton 2011: 71). Implicit research addresses 'prenoetic' processes (Gallagher 2006: 6), such as kinesthetic empathy and other forms of simulated communication via the mirror neuron system (Gallese 2009) and, certainly, other forms of transformational consciousness. For examples of this kind of research on embodied cognition, see Gallagher 2006; Reynolds and Reason 2012; and Jola, Ehrenberg and Reynolds 2012.

2　For reviews on task-based/constraint-led research from the human movement science perspective, consult Davids, Button and Bennett (2008); Davids, Button and Newell (2006); and Serrien, Ivry and Swinnen (2007).

3　On the other hand, dance is often used to 'explain' complex concepts. For example, Wake Forest University dance professor Christina Soriano collaborated with chemistry professor Dr. Rebecca Alexander in a course called 'Movement and the Molecular'. This course brought non-dance students together to express complex concepts from biology and chemistry through dance: see http://news.wfu.edu/2012/04/27/the-science-of-dance/.

4　As one dance artist aptly put it: 'I want a definition of dance that is big enough for my practice.' Courtesy of Celeste Miller, notebook entry (with permission), 'Contemporary Body Practices', Hollins/ADF Masters in Fine Arts Program, Durham, NC, 2009.

5　Sheets-Johnstone suggests that dynamics are essentially modes of animation (Sheets-Johnstone 2009: 483). They anchor coordination in a temporal rather than a purely spatial concept of mind (ibid. 483). Based on highly complex principles from theoretical physics, mathematics and ecological psychology, dynamical systems theory proposes that qualitative changes in motor behavior emerge out of the naturally developing dynamic properties of the motor system and coordinative structures (Kelso 1995; Kugler, Kelso and Turvey 1982; Thelen and Smith 1996).

6　Daniel Nagrin explores this concept in his book *The Six Questions* (1997) where he provides explorations into dance meaning and context through linking words and movement. I have pitched these basic questions from the perspective of a news reporter (Covello 2003).

7　Task constraints have been looked at primarily in sport, focusing on, for example, the rules of a game, contextual sources of information, performance space, equipment and the number of individuals involved in the activity. In addition, personal, environmental and sociocultural constraints shape the way a player responds in a given situation. See Chow et al. 2006 and 2007; Renshaw et al. 2010; and Renshaw et al. 2012, for more detailed reviews of the different categories of constraints.

8　Constraints are categorized as environmental, organismic and task-specific (Newell 1986). Human system constraints are musculoskeletal, immunological, cognitive and more. Structural constraints including height, weight, strength and flexibility impact on individual kinetic and kinematic variations in movement and the development of skill. These constraints narrow the infinite number of movement possibilities (degrees of freedom) to help simplify the organizational components of the task at hand. Psychophysical constraints also support movement performance (Davids, Button, and Bennett 2008). These include awareness and attention, 'intentions, emotions, perception, decision-making and memory' (Glazier and Davids 2009: 20). Last, there are external (or environmental) constraints, including light, surface, texture etc. Take the example of brushing your teeth: the height of the sink, the distance of your face from the basin and the mirror, the angle of your toothbrush, the water temperature, the taste of the toothpaste…all these constrain movement dynamics.

9　See Chapter 6 on 'attending' for a fuller explanation of cognitive load.

10　Iteration is a process by which repetition yields variations that enable reaching the desired goal/target or aim of a particular task. Although used largely within mathematics, computing and robotics, iteration has been adapted in human movement science and self-regulation theory to imply variable means of goal attainment. It has also been adapted in dance to suggest reciprocal processes of practice and reflection, re-entry and re-investment in developing movement material. For explication, see http://portal.unesco.org/culture/es/files/40494/12668597373Dance_education.pdf/Dance%2Beducation.pdf.

11 Although not explicitly framed as task-based analyses, a number of studies on cognition in dancemaking exemplify this approach. We could not report the results of all of these here. For one of the earliest examples, see Stevens et al. 2003. This dance–science collaboration pioneered a model for dance-specific movement creation, based on the Geneplore model of creative cognition (Finke, Ward and Smith 1996), which captured both 'generative and exploratory cognitive processes' (ibid.: 317). More recent studies expanded the use of motion-capture tools, including video- and other motion-capture technology, choreographic field notes, interviews (with both choreographer and dancers), structured (guided) journaling or diaries (both structured and unstructured reflections), neuropsychological batteries, and neurologic imaging/recordings, such as fMRI scanning and transcranial magnetic stimulation or EEG recordings. See Brown, Martinez and Parsons 2006; Nielsen and Cohen 2008; Kirsh 2009; Kirsh 2011; Jola 2010.

12 View summaries of various studies on choreographer Wayne McGregor's research on imagery at http://www.choreocog.net/. Also, consult the study by Kirsh et al. 2009, http://adrenaline.ucsd.edu/Kirsh/publications.html.

Chapter 4

Reframing Embodiment

Cognition is embodied insofar as it emerges not from an intricately unfolding cognitive program but from a dynamic dance in which body, perception, and world guide each other's steps.

(Lawrence Shapiro 2010: 61)

Overview

For centuries, western scholars maintained a strict division between mind and body. By the later part of the twentieth century, the topic of phenomenological embodiment had gained considerable currency in academic circles, as well as in dance and somatic studies. During this period, cognitive science also aligned with phenomenology, giving rise to of the concept of embodied cognition. Scientist Humberto Maturana and protégé Francisco Varela evolved a theory of embodied cognition in the 1970s. Varela continued to advance this theory through the 1990s, along with his colleague, philosopher Evan Thompson. Embodied cognitive theory continues to pose challenges to classical cognitive science and influence other disciplines, including dance. In light of the current exchange between dance and science, this chapter revisits *embodiment* in dance. The chapter provides a brief history of the origin of embodied cognitive theory and points to its continuing relevance within dancemaking.

Focusing in…

- Define embodiment in dancemaking. From where do you derive your definition?
- Why is a context-specific term for embodiment important for dance research?
- How did the term 'embodied cognition' evolve within cognitive science? State the embodied hypothesis.

Experiential prelude

Before reading on, take a moment to become more present. *How* did you become more present? What processes did you invoke? What sensations surfaced in the foreground of your attention? What sensations awakened you to animate alive-ness? How does this current state exemplify being *more embodied* than you were moments ago? What effect is this shift having on your experience of this moment? What effect is it having on your attention as you read? Do you perceive yourself and the room differently now? If you are a dancer (or other performing artist), how do you prepare to become more embodied? Why is this change necessary? What starts the process? Is it an *awareness* or *intention* to become more embodied? How do you start? What enables the process to continue? If you pursue any mindfully embodied practice, what routine do you follow – or is your approach improvisational? How do you *customize* an embodiment practice to suit a particular situation in performance – dancing, singing, lecturing etc. What needs does this practice meet?

Introduction

The *Oxford English Dictionary* (2012) defines embodiment as 'a tangible or visible form of an idea, quality or feeling'. *Embodiment* suggests a phenomenal quality, the 'epitome', 'incarnation' or 'incorporation' of something material. As a noun, embodiment is an expression of qualities of *being*, of having or existing in, a biological body. Embodiment also is 'the representation or expression of something in such a form'. As a verb, *embodying* suggests agency – the capacity and capability of human beings to act intelligently and expressively through their bodies.

Today, the term *embodiment* circulates widely among dancemakers. At the same time, the term lacks specificity. Like a chameleon, the term tends to change its colors depending on context. The ambiguity remaining around this term renders it 'at risk of losing explanatory power' (Warburton 2011: 66). *How* do dancers become embodied to serve artistic purposes? By what processes or actions do dancers become *more* embodied? Arriving at context-specific definitions of embodiment, bears on the integrity of praxis research.

From the 1960s through the 1990s, embodiment became an intellectual buzzword in sociocultural, artistic and scientific circles (Bresler 2004). Through cross-disciplinary encounters, scholars began to shift their views away from strictly dualist concepts of body and mind (O'Donovan-Anderson 1996). Dance scholars grounded their explanations of embodied dance experience largely in phenomenological and sociocultural theory (Sheets-Johnstone 1981; Fraleigh 1996; 2004; Ashead-Landsdale 1988; Desmond 2003; van Manen 2007; Dragon 2008 – to name a few authors tackling the subject within dance). Issues of body, embodiment and inter-subjectivity brought dance into alignment with the humanities as well as with somatic praxis (Green 2007; Schusterman 2008). This rich archive of scholarship contributed significantly to an understanding of body identity, power relations, aesthetics, societal and ritualistic practices and more (Fraleigh 1996; Parviainen 1998; Sheets-Johnstone 2011). To date, phenomenology remains one critical avenue crucial for gaining an intellectual understanding of 'embodied knowing' (Rouhiainen 2007). This branch of philosophy remains pivotal both in shaping the learning and explicating the meaning of dance experience. Further, it helps align dance with contemporary scientific theory on embodiment.

Cognitive science also engaged in the intellectual flurry around embodiment. While the roots of embodied *cognition* can be traced back to the 1970s, the concept remains radical today.[1] Major contributors to the original theory include Chilean biologist and cognitive neuroscientist Francisco Varela (1946–2001) and his mentor Humberto Maturana. Between the early 1970s until he died (2004), Varela argued for a theory in which the biological, sense-making body was *constitutive* of cognition (Shapiro 2010). Varela, along with his colleagues, philosopher Evan Thompson and cognitive scientist Eleanor Rosch, coined the phrase 'embodied cognition' and evolved an embodiment hypothesis (Varela, Thompson and Rosch 1991). From their viewpoint, bodily experience is not merely *associated* with cognition; rather, lived experience is *foundational* to consciousness, mind and thought. Although embodiment is *of* the body,[2] the degree to which the body actually gives rise to thinking remains at the center of the debate.

This chapter revisits embodiment in dancemaking within the context of embodied cognitive theory. We provide a historical overview of the emergence of embodiment theory within cognitive science. Reviewing the origins of embodiment science enriches our understanding of the scope of cognitive studies.

Locating embodiment within dance

Phenomenological embodiment is an existential birthright. It is the expression or manifestation of humanness through experience (Brown and Reid 2006). Embodiment is 'ontological attunement' (Block and Kissell 2001: 2). More than something inherited, learned or cultivated, it enables '...the subjective source or inter-subjective ground of experience' (Csordas 1999: 143). As embodied beings, humans are 'thoughtful, intelligent, and practical' (Brown and Reid 2006: 179). They are also social (Gallese 2006: 6). Humans are 'endowed with a sense of coherence, agency, affectivity, and continuity...[with] a readiness (or unreadiness) to come into relationship and interact with others' (Stern 2000: 44–45). Embodiment affords the capacity and capability to intuit, infer, empathize, mimic and be at one with others.

Embodiment is not *about* the body, but rather about the generative power of movement. From the perspective of neuroscience, intention is an 'action ontology' (Metzinger and Gallese 2003: 549), the way ideas translate into action. This is a pivotal concept in dance. To be *em*-bodied is to be empowered to act. Embodiment is not a state or trait that emerges from the brain or the body alone (Sheets-Johnstone 2009), but from their confluence in creating experience.[3] Dance enlivens the material body through 'embodied knowing' (Rouhiainen 2007; de Lima 2013). 'Embodied knowing is the ability to interact with a thought or an experience holistically that involves the integrated power network of the total person' (Block and Kissell 2001: 6).

Dance is a particular *kind* of embodied knowing (Rouhiainen 2007; Klemola 1991; Fraleigh 1996; Noland 2009). Becoming more *intentionally* embodied (as dancers do) facilitates artistic communication by rendering the dancing body more transparent (van Manen 2007; Fraleigh 1996).[4] The dancer's primary intention is for the chosen movement dynamics to be seen and communicated as a shared art form (Jola 2010; Block and Kissell 2001). Dancing intends toward deeper embodied connections to self (soma) in order to become more outwardly expressive (Clarke, Cramer and Müller 2010). Through praxis, dancers prepare the body 'to invite being seen' (attributed to Deborah Hay, quoted in Clarke, Cramer and Müller 2010: 202). In practice, the body becomes 'permeable' and 'see-able' (Clarke, Kramer and Müller 2010: 202). In constructing an embodied aesthetic, all systems are engaged: intellectual, emotional and physical. Why would it be important for dancemakers 'to create movement with intent?' (Green 2010: 31). Intention contextualizes dance beyond its general aesthetic aims, specifies its tasks and its communicative goals and provides insight into the cognitive processes underlying choice and decision-making.

In this way, dance goes beyond ordinary everyday embodiment toward something more extra-ordinary, toward an 'integrated motional style of being' (Rouhiainen 2003: 328). Through dancing, movers shift from engaging at the surface to engaging with deeper levels of experience (Garrett Brown et al. 2012). 'In a well-done dance, the self is lived beyond personal finitude and limitations. The body is experienced as all of self and more than self' (Fraleigh 1996: 34). Each moment of movement is an expression of attunement to dynamics that 'give tangible form to ideas' (Preston-Dunlop and Sanchez-Colberg 2002: 3). In one stroke, embodiment in dance deals a deathblow to dualism.

Dance thus affords a sense of immediacy between thought and action, a 'hyper-reflection' in which thought and movement 'form a partnership' (Kozel 2007: 22). The experience is immersive and unmediated. No intermediary images or representations, no internal schema, no motor plan or mental calculation of mind, separates the dancer from the dance (Sheets-Johnstone 2009). This unmediated experience in dance arguably is one of the largest hurdles in finding compatibility in science research (Krasnow 2005; deLahunta, Barnard and McGregor 2009). This hurdle has been eased somewhat by a number of theoretical and technical advances on contemporary themes in science. One of these themes is embodied cognition.

Francisco Varela and embodied cognition

One of the earliest theories of embodied cognition was formulated in the 1970s by biologist Humberto Maturana and his protégé (biologist, immunologist and cognitive neuroscientist) Francisco Varela (Maturana and Varela 1980; 1992). Many cognitive scientists advanced theories of embodied cognition in second- and third-generation cognitive science, such as linguists

George Lakoff and Mark Johnson (Lakoff and Johnson 1980; 1999). Varela was by far the most influential and radical of the early proponents of embodied cognition, however. While no one person can be given full credit for causing a paradigm shift, the link between embodiment and consciousness is most strongly associated with his work (Rudrauf et al. 2003).

The concept of embodiment posed a significant challenge to traditional theory in cognitive science (Shapiro 2010). Embodied cognitive theory posed an alternative to dualistic divisions between the mental and the physical (Fuchs and De Jaegher 2009). Within classical cognitive science, it was inconceivable to place bodily experience as causal to cognition. Varela's theories helped shift the cognitive paradigm from a computational theory of cognition toward an experiential one.

Varela was a biologist, immunologist, philosopher, cognitive scientist, mathematician and overall Renaissance man (Rudrauf et al. 2003). Moreover, Varela's approach to describing phenomena such as consciousness, thought and mind was rooted in pragmatic and experiential studies. Varela also maintained an extensive commitment to Tibetan Buddhist practice. He derived his view of reality from his extensive investment in biological complexity, self-organization and Buddhist epistemology, rather than from information science and engineering (Zahn 2011). He assigned the biological body a central role in shaping thought. First-person experience should be the starting point for understanding cognition. He stated: '[D]isciplined first-person accounts should be an integral element of the validation of a neurobiological proposal, and not merely coincidental or heuristic information' (Varela 1996: 344). His views resonated deeply with Somatics and other pragmatic approaches to conscious change. His legacy continues to inspire researchers to probe the basic tenets of cognitive science (Shapiro 2010; Gallagher and Zahavi 2012). During his brief life, Varela wrote more than 180 articles and was the sole author of ten books (editing and collaborating on many more). Topics ranged from theoretical and natural biology, immunology, neurology and neuropathology (epilepsy) to cognitive science, mathematics and phenomenology, including the epistemology of science and Buddhist spirituality.

His ideas on living systems first came to prominence in the late 1960s, when he and Maturana developed a construct for a biology of consciousness and cognition: autopoiesis (Maturana and Varela 1980). Autopoiesis is based on the assumption that there is no preordained reality. Instead, living organisms *enact*, or bring forth, reality. Autopoiesis incorporated elements from dynamic systems theory and mathematics. Living organisms are autopoietic gestalts. They are intelligent cellular systems acting autonomously in creating a world. Living organisms are embedded in space-time through ongoing cycles of internal regulation and sensory attunement (Rudrauf et al. 2003). Living organisms are 'self-maintaining, self-regulating, self-producing and self-distinguishing' (Froese 2011: 214).

Autopoietic systems, therefore, are *cognitive*. Humans acquire knowledge through their *situated living bodies* (Colombetti 2010). Cognition arises from the dynamic sensorimotor coupling between organism and environment – immediate, intimate and reciprocal

(Thompson and Varela 2001; de Bruin and Kastner 2012). Both body and brain are needed in the co-creation of reality (Varela 1979). The brain governs plasticity, connectivity and complexity. At the same time, the brain should not be privileged. Reality cannot exist independently of the organism; the brain cannot represent an accurate model of that world before it acts. The focus of theories of cognition, then, should be on experience – not on computational and representational mechanisms.

Varela coined the term 'embodied cognition'. He co-authored *The Embodied Mind* (1991), with his colleagues, philosopher Evan Thompson and cognitive psychologist Eleanor Rosch. Here, the authors attempt to redirect the cognitive sciences away from mechanistic computational models. This book is considered 'the *ur* text' for embodied cognitive theory (Shapiro 2010: 52). The content aligns with the phenomenological perspectives of Edmund Husserl and Maurice Merleau-Ponty.[5] It is a classic for advancing a neuro-phenomenological theory of cognition that included the following tenets:

- *Mind* is grounded in the evolution and mutual interaction of the physical body with the environment.
- Embodiment is grounded in the sense-making physiological body we possess, which also constrains us.
- Cognition depends upon the actions of a goal-directed, intentional body in the coupling of perception and action.
- The inter-subjective body is social, extending beyond boundaries of the brain and anatomy.[6]

Toward a neuro-phenomenological methodology

Varela and his colleagues called for a revolution in cognitive science, rather than a mere set of reforms (Rudrauf et al. 2003). This revolution would place first-person experience squarely in the center of cognitive theory.[7] In his final decade, Varela created a structured methodology for the study of consciousness and first-person experience called 'neuro-phenomenology' (Varela 1996). Neuro-phenomenology is the study of the 'irreducible nature of conscious experience' (Varela 1996: 334). 'Phenomenology is anchored to the careful description, analysis and interpretation of lived experience' (Thompson 2007:16). Experience is *'die unhintergehbarkeit'*, the 'ungobehindable' (Varela 1996: 394). Here, living experience – not dualism or idealism – defines reality (Zahn 2005; Zahn 2011). Experience is not a biological feature of the body but the result of interaction (Thompson 2007). Experience is a gestalt – embodied, unfragmented, situated and communicative. In essence, seven 'E's' define experience: embodied, embedded, enmeshed, emergent, extended, enactive and empathic (Gallagher; Stewart 2010; Reynolds and Reason 2012).

Varela believed this prelude to a methodology to be an important step within cognitive neuroscience in enabling a rigorous examination of first-person experience (Varela 1977; Thompson and Varela 2001). Drawing from phenomenology and dynamic systems theory, Varela and Thompson went on to design a method to substantiate embodied cognition.[8] Utilizing brain-imaging to map large-scale neural dynamics, they analyzed dynamical patterns of neural substrates of conscious experience (Thompson and Varela 2001). Since his untimely death in 2004, a number of scientific studies have shown initial success at studying first-person experience that have gone beyond the introspective approach that Varela adapted from Buddhism (Gallagher and Zahavi 2012). The current scientific generation continues to research embodied cognition (Stewart 2010; Clark 1997; Shapiro 2010). Using contemporary methods of technology and digital media, scientists have designed many topical studies on embodied cognition – action and agency, intentionality, the self and inter-subjectivity, kinesthetic empathy and social cognition (Gallagher and Zahavi 2012) (see Box 4.1).

Embodiment science – a continuing challenge

Embodied cognitive theory opened the door to a science of personal experience (Varela and Shear 1999).[9] To advance Varela's model is to challenge Cartesian dualistic models of research and reductionist paradigms that fragment holistic experience. Varela was a pioneer in advancing both a theory of embodied cognition and a methodology for examining experience.[10] While Varela shifted the paradigm within cognitive science, critics continue to challenge the validity of his legacy (Sheets-Johnstone 2011; McGann and Jaegher 2009). And, science remains confronted by the ineffable nature of embodied experience (Borgdorff 2009).[11] Models of cognition may exist, but scientists still need to adequately describe many experiences and cognitive states. Experience remains elusive, tangential, transient and evanescent, subject to fluctuations in attention and memory (Petitmengin 2001). While experience is 'intimate and directly accessible...[we are, at the same time] 'never fully...self-aware' (Petitmengin 2007: 7). Experience may be unfiltered or it may be edited, censored and otherwise suppressed, so that deficiencies can go unnoticed and unobserved (Petitmengin 2001; 2007). Further, experiential phenomena are not located anywhere – it is corporeally resonant knowledge that is tied to its meaningful context (Zahavi 2010).

The phenomenological challenge within dancemaking lies along this spectrum of being able to capture actual embodied experience (Rouhiainen 2012). Dancers need to go beyond simply calling an experience 'embodied'. The phenomena of dance, i.e., the 'things themselves', are not objects, things or states of being, 'but precisely *moving* phenomena that are *movingly* experienced – 'dynamic, processual happenings' (Sheets-Johnstone 2011: 456). This challenge also begs for terms of embodiment that are satisfactory to dancers and scientists alike (Sheets-Johnstone 2009; Warburton 2011; deLahunta 2013).

Explorations for this chapter appear in Appendix II.

Box 4.1: Sample of neuroscientific studies on experience

Farrer, C., Franck, N., Georgieff, N., Frith, D., Decety, J. and Jeannerod, M. (2003), 'Modulating the experience of agency: A positron emission tomography study', *NeuroImage*, 18, pp. 324–33.

Farrer, C. and Frith, C. (2002), 'Experiencing oneself vs. another person as being the cause of an action: The neural correlates of the experience of agency', *NeuroImage*, 15, pp. 596–603.

Frith, C. (2002), 'How can we share experiences?', *Trends in Cognitive Sciences*, 6: 9, p. 374.

Le Van Quyen, M. and Petitmengin, C. (2002), 'Neuronal dynamics and conscious experience: An example of reciprocal causation before epileptic seizures', *Phenomenology and the Cognitive Sciences*, 1: 2, pp. 169–80.

Lutz, A. and Thompson, E. (2003), 'Neurophenomenology integrating subjective experience and brain dynamics in the neuroscience of consciousness', *Journal of Consciousness Studies*, 10: 9–10, pp. 31–52.

Myin, E. and O'Regan, J.K. (2002), 'Perceptual consciousness, access to modality and skill theories', *Journal of Consciousness Studies*, 9: 1, pp. 27–45.

Nahab et al. (2011), 'The neural processes underlying self-agency', *Cerebral Cortex*, 21, pp. 48–55.

References

Adshead-Lansdale, J. (ed.) (1988), *Dance Analysis: Theory and Practice*, Lincoln, UK: Dance Books Ltd.

Block, B. and Kissell, J. (2001), 'The dance: Essence of embodiment', *Theoretical Medicine*, 22, pp. 5–15.

Borgdorff, H. (2009), *Artistic Research Within the Fields of Science*, Bergen: Kunsthøgskolen.

Borghi, A. and Cimatti, F. (2010), 'Embodied cognition and beyond: Acting and sensing the body', *Neuropsychologia*, 48: 3, pp. 763–73.

Bresler, L. (2004), *Knowing Bodies, Moving Minds: Towards Embodied Teaching and Learning*, London: Kluwer Academic Publishers.

Brown, L. and Reid, D. (2006), 'Embodied cognition: Somatic markers, purposes and emotional orientations', *Educational Studies in Mathematics*, 63: 2, pp. 179–92.

Bruner, J.S. (1962), *The Purposes of Education*, Cambridge, MA: Harvard University Press.

Chalmers, D.J. (1995), 'Facing up to the problem of consciousness', *Journal of Consciousness Studies*, 2: 3, pp. 200–19.

Chalmers, D. (1999), 'Materialism and the metaphysics of modality', *Philosophy and Phenomenological Research*, 59: 2, pp. 473–96.

Clark, A. (1997), *Being There: Putting Mind, World, and Body Back Together*, Cambridge, MA: MIT Press.

Clarke, G., Cramer, F. and Müller, G. (2010), 'Minding motion' in I. Diehl and F. Lampert (eds.), *Dance Techniques 2010*, Leipzig: Henschel Verlag, pp. 199–29.

Colombetti, G. (2010), 'Enaction, sense-making and emotion' in J. Stewart, O. Gapenne and E. Di Paolo (eds.), *Enaction: Towards a New Paradigm for Cognitive Science*, Cambridge, MA: MIT Press, pp. 145–64.

Csordas, T. (1999), 'Embodiment and cultural phenomenology' in G. Weiss and H. Honi (eds.), *Perspectives on Embodiment*, London: Routledge, pp. 143–62.

de Bruin, L.C. and Kästner, L. (2012), 'Dynamic embodied cognition', *Phenomenology and the Cognitive Sciences*, 11, pp. 541–63.

deLahunta, S. (2013), 'Publishing choreographic ideas', in E. Boxberger and G. Wittmann (eds.), *pARTnering Documentation: Approaching Dance, Heritage*, Culture. 3rd Dance Education Biennae 2012 Frankfurt am Main. Munchen, DE: Epodium Verlag, pp. 18–25.

deLahunta, S., Barnard, P. and McGregor, W. (2009), 'Augmenting choreography: Using insights and inspiration from science' in J. Butterworth and L. Wildschut (eds.), *Contemporary Choreography: A Critical Reader*, New York, NY: Routledge, pp. 431–38.

de Lima, C. (2013), 'Trans-meaning – Dance as an embodied technology of perception', *Journal of Dance and Somatic Practices*, 5: 1, pp. 17–30.

Desmond, J. (ed.) (2003), *Meaning in Motion: New Cultural Studies of Dance*. Durham, NC: Duke University Press.

Di Paolo, E., Rohde, M. and De Jaegher, H. (2010), 'Horizons for the enactive mind: Values, social interaction, and play' in J. Stewart, O. Gapenne and E. Di Paolo (eds.), *Enaction: Towards a New Paradigm for Cognitive Science*, Cambridge, MA: MIT Press, pp. 33–88.

Dragon, D. (2008), *Toward Embodied Education, 1850s–2007: Historical, Cultural, Theoretical and Methodological Perspectives Impacting Somatic Education in United States Higher Education Dance*, Doctoral Dissertation, Temple University, Philadelphia PA, UMI number 3326321.

Fraleigh, S.H. (1996), *Dance and the Lived Body: A Descriptive Aesthetics*, Pittsburgh, PA: University of Pittsburgh Press.

Fraleigh, S.H. (1999), 'Family resemblance' in S. Fraleigh and P. Hanstein (eds.), *Researching Dance: Evolving Modes of Inquiry*, Pittsburgh, PA: University of Pittsburgh Press.

Fraleigh, S.H. (2004), *Dancing Identity: Metaphysics in Motion*, Pittsburgh, PA: University of Pittsburgh Press.

Froese, T. (2011), 'From second-order cybernetics to enactive cognitive science: Varela's turn from epistemology to phenomenology', *Systems Research and Behavioral Science*, 28: 6, pp. 631–38.

Fuchs, T. and De Jaegher, H. (2009), 'Enactive intersubjectivity: Participatory sense-making and mutual incorporation', *Phenomenology and the Cognitive Sciences*, 8: 4, pp. 465–86.

Gallagher, S. (2007), 'Cognition: Embodied, Embedded, Enacted, Extended', Interdisciplinary Conference, Orlando, FL: University of Central Florida.

Gallagher, S. and Zahavi, D. (2012), *The Phenomenological Mind*, 2nd edn, New York, NY: Routledge.

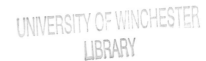

Gallese, V. (2006), 'Mirror neurons and intentional attunement: Commentary on Olds', *Journal of the American Psychoanalytic Association*, 54: 1, pp. 47–57.

Garrett-Brown, N., Kipp, C., Pollard, N. and Voris, A. (2012), 'Everything is at once: Reflections on embodied photography and collaborative process', *Journal of Dance and Somatic Practices* 3: 1–2, pp. 75–84.

Green, D. (2010), *Choreographing From Within: Developing the Habit of Inquiry as an Artist*, Champaign, IL: Human Kinetics Press.

Green, J. (2007), 'Student bodies: Dance pedagogy and the soma', *Springer International Handbook of Research in Arts Education*, 16, pp. 1119–3533.

Hanna, T. (1973), 'The project of Somatology', *Journal of Humanistic Psychology*, 13: 3, pp. 3–13.

Jola, C. (2010), 'Research and choreography' in B. Bläsing, M. Puttke and T. Schack (eds.), *The Neurocognition of Dance: Mind, Movement and Motor Skills*, New York, NY: Psychology Press.

Klemola, T. (1991),'Dance and embodiment', *Ballet International*, 1: 1, pp. 71–80.

Kozel, S. (2007), *Closer: Performance, Technologies, Phenomenology*, Cambridge, MA: MIT Press.

Krasnow, D. (2005), 'Sustaining the dance artist: Barriers to communication between educators, artists, and researchers' in K. Vincs (ed.), *Conference Proceedings: Dance Rebooted: Initialing the Grid*, Ausdance National Australia 2004.

Lakoff, G. and Johnson, M. (1980), *Metaphors We Live By*, Chicago, IL: University of Chicago Press.

Lakoff, G. and Johnson, M. (1999), *Philosophy in the Flesh: The Embodied Mind and Its Challenge to Western Thought*, New York, NY: Basic Books.

Levin, D. (1985), *The Body's Recollection of Being: Phenomenological Psychology and the Deconstruction of Nihilism*, Boston, MA: Routledge & Kegan Paul.

McGann, M. and Jaegher, H. (2009), 'Self-other contingencies: Enacting social perception', *Phenomenology and the Cognitive Sciences*, 8: 4, pp. 417–37.

Maturana, H. and Varela, F. (1980), *Autopoiesis and Cognition: The Realization of the Living*, London: Riedl.

Maturana, H. and Varela, F. (1992), *The Tree of Knowledge: The Biological Roots of Human Understanding* (rev. edn), Boston, MA: Shambala.

Metzinger, T. and Gallese, V. (2003), 'The emergence of a shared action ontology: Building blocks for a theory', *Consciousness and Cognition*, 12: 4, pp. 549–71.

Noland, C. (2009), *Agency and Embodiment: Performing Gestures/Producing Culture*, Cambridge, MA: Harvard University Press.

O'Donovan-Anderson, J. (1996), *The Incorporated Self: Interdisciplinary Perspectives on Embodiment*, Lanham, MD: Rowman and Littlefield.

Parviainen, J. (1998), 'Bodies moving and moved: A phenomenological analysis of the dancing subject and the cognitive and ethical values of dance art', Doctoral Thesis. Tampere, FI: Tampere University Press.

Parviainen, J. (2002), 'Epistemology reflections on dance', *Dance Research Journal*, 34: 1, pp. 11–18.

Petitmengin, C. (2001), *L'expérience Intuitive. Préface de Francisco Varela*, Paris: L'Harmattan.

Petitmengin, C. (2007), 'Towards the source of thoughts: The gestural and transmodal dimension of lived experience', *Journal of Consciousness Studies*, 14: 3, pp. 54–82.

Petitmengin, C. (2009), *Ten years of Viewing From Within: The Legacy of Francisco Varela*, Charlottesville, VA: Imprint Academic.

Preston-Dunlop, V. and Sanchez-Colberg, A. (2002), *Dance and the Performative: A Choreological Perspective – Laban and Beyond*, London: Verve.

Reynolds, D. and Reason, M. (2012), *Kinesthetic Empathy in Creative and Cultural Contexts*, Chicago, IL: University of Chicago Press.

Rouhiainen, L. (2003), *Living Transformative Lives. Finnish Freelance Dance Artists*, Helsinki: Theatre Academy.

Rouhiainen, L. (2007), 'Ways of Knowing in Dance and Art', *Acta Scenica*, 19, Helsinki: Teaterhögskolan.

Rouhiainen, L. (2012), 'An investigation into facilitating the work of the independent contemporary dancer through somatic psychology', *Journal of Dance and Somatic Practices*, 3: 1–2, pp. 43–59.

Rudrauf, D., Lutz, A., Cosmelli, D., Lachaux, J. and Le Van Ouven, M. (2003), 'From autopoiesis to neurophenmenology: Francisco Varela's exploration of the biophysics of being', *Biological Research*, 36: 1, pp. 27–65.

Schusterman, R. (2008), *Body Consciousness: A Philosophy of Mindfulness and Somaesthetics*, New York, NY: Cambridge University Press.

Shapiro, L. (2010), *Embodied Cognition*, New York, NY: Routledge.

Sheets-Johnstone, M. (1981), 'Thinking in movement', *The Journal of Aesthetics and Art Criticism*, 39: 4, pp. 399–407.

Sheets-Johnstone, M. (2009), *The Corporeal Turn: An Interdisciplinary Reader*, Exeter, UK: Imprint Academic.

Sheets-Johnstone, M. (2011), *The Primacy of Movement*, expanded 2nd edn, Philadelphia, PA: John Benjamins Publishing Company.

Stern, D. (2000), *The Interpersonal World of the Infant: A View From Psychoanalysis and Developmental Psychology*, Philadelphia, PA: Basic Books.

Stewart, J. (2010), 'Foundational issues in enaction as a paradigm for cognitive science: From the origin of life to consciousness and writing' in J. Stewart, O. Gapenne, E. Di Paolo (eds.), *Enaction: Toward a New Paradigm for Cognitive Science*, London: MIT Press.

Stewart, J., Gapenne, O. and Di Paolo, E. (eds.), *Enaction: Toward a New Paradigm for Cognitive Science*, London: MIT Press.

Thelen, E. (2008), 'Self-organization in developmental processes: Can systems approach work?' in M.H. Johnson, Y. Funakata and R.O. Gilmore (eds.), *Brain Development and Cognition: A Reader*, Wiley online library, http://onlinelibrary.wiley.com/doi/10.1002/9780470753507.ch18/summary. Accessed 14 October 2013.

Thompson, E. and Varela, F. (2001), 'Radical embodiment: Neural dynamics and consciousnesses', *Trends in the Cognitive Sciences*, 5: 10, pp. 418–25.

Thompson, E. (ed.) (2001), *Between Ourselves: Second-Person Issues in the Study of Consciousness*, Charlottesville, VA: Imprint Academic.

Thompson, E. (2007), *Mind in Life: Biology, Phenomenology, and the Sciences of Mind*, New York, NY: Belknap Press.

Van Manen, M. (2007), 'Phenomenology of practice', *Phenomenology and Practice*, 1: 1, pp. 11–30.

Varela, F.J. (1977), 'The nervous system as a closed network', *Brain Theory Newsletter*, 2, pp. 66–67.

Varela, F. (1979), *Principles of Biological Autonomy*, New York, NY: Elsevier North Holland.

Varela, F., Thompson, E. and Rosch, E. (1991), *The Embodied Mind: Cognitive Science and Human Experience*, Cambridge, MA: MIT Press.

Varela, F. (1996), 'Neurophenomenology: A methodological remedy for the hard problem', *Journal of Consciousness Studies*, 3: 4, pp. 330–49.

Varela, F. and Shear, J. (1999), 'First-person methodologies: What, Why, How?' in F.J. Varela and J. Shear (eds.), *The View From Within: First-Person Approaches to the Study of Consciousness*, Exeter, UK: Imprint Academic, pp. 2–14.

Warburton, E. (2011), 'Of Meanings and movements: Re-languaging embodiment in dance phenomenology and cognition', *Dance Research Journal*, 43: 2, pp. 65–83.

Zahavi, D. (2010), 'Husserl and the "absolute" ' in C. Ierna, H. Jacobs and F. Mattens (eds.), *Philosophy, Phenomenology, Sciences: Essays in Commemoration of Husserl, Phaenomenologica* vol. 200, Dordrecht, NL: Springer, pp. 71–92.

Zahn, R. (2005), 'Francisco Varela and the gesture of awareness: A new direction in cognitive science and its relevance to the Alexander Technique', *Proceedings of the 7th International Congress of the F.M. Alexander Technique*, University of Oxford, UK, August 2004.

Zahn, R. (2011), 'The Embodied mind: The domain of second-person psychophysical experts', *Proceedings of the 9th International Congress of the F.M. Alexander Technique*, Lugano, Switzerland, August 2011 (unpublished).

Notes

1 Cognitive science continues, however, to evolve various definitions for embodied cognition with the development of robotics, virtual reality and artificial intelligence. See Borghi and Cimatti 2010 and Gallagher and Zahavi 2012 for further explanation. At the same time, critics claim that scientific interpretations of embodiment remain dualistic. Dance phenomenologist Maxine Sheets-Johnstone writes: 'When we strip the lexical band-aid *"embodiment"* off the more than 350 year-old wound inflicted by the Cartesian split of mind and body, we find *animation*, the foundational dimension of the living' (Maxine Sheets-Johnstone 2011: 453).

2 For dance scholar Sheets-Johnstone (2009), the phrase *embodied movement* or embodied cognition is a tautology. Human beings are born into moving bodies and are therefore embodied. She argues that movement is the manifestation of a relating body whose very nature is embodiment. Simply having a body means we belong to ourselves and to our world making in ways that are integrally 'embodied'. The moving, sensate self is enmeshed in the act of incorporating and making a world. Our experience is grounded in the spatiotemporal and kinetic/energetic real-time elements of movement

(Sheets-Johnstone 2011: 145, 147). Experience, therefore, is 'first and foremost by way of the tactile-kinesthetic body' and its resonant dynamics (Sheets-Johnstone 2011: 231 – after Gibson). Embodiment supports agency, affectivity and the dynamics of movement. It is not a bodily 'attribute' or 'role.' A state of non-embodiment is 'death' (ibid. 91–92). An animate body is by its very nature *embodied*. In a similar vein, dance phenomenologist Sondra Fraleigh asks the question, 'what is the opposite of dance? Lassitude? (Fraleigh 1999: 4).

3 Movement brings about 'a systems holistic experience [of] relationship with our selves, others, and the world' (Levin 1985: 295). To paraphrase motor development scientist Esther Thelen (2008), '...crying exists neither in the organism nor in the environment, but only in their confluence'.

4 Dance arguably is not always *intentional*. It also can be, spontaneous and improvisational, issuing from non-consciously directed sources of embodied knowledge. Equally, dance arguably is not always *expressive*. Here, we use it in the context of dance destined for expressive (theatrical) performance – regardless of the context of the theater. Further, dance is not always performative (intended for performance). Here, we use the term 'performative' according to its roots. Perform (etymology) – c.1300, 'carry into effect, fulfill, discharge', via Anglo-Fr. *performir*, altered (by influence of O.Fr. *forme* 'form') from O.Fr. *parfornir* 'to do, carry out, finish, accomplish', from *par-* 'completely' + *fornir* 'to provide'. We also use the term 'performative' rather than 'expressive' to distinguish dance from other forms of physical expression (conscious and non-conscious). See http://www.etymonline.com/index.php?term=perform.

5 Phenomenology aims not for a *description* of experience (the *what* of experience), but rather 'attempts to capture the invariant structure of experience'. This brings the field into alliance with science (Gallagher and Zahavi 2012: 28). For Varela and his colleagues, the phenomenological tradition finds its validity in 'its ability to transform progressively our lived experience and self-understanding' (Varela, Thompson and Rosch 1991: xix). The perspective that worldly experience is constitutive of cognition remains radical within some circles. Experience, Varela stated, 'at once frees the concept of cognition from an abstract, functionalist model of the dis-embodied brain, while on the other hand demands a rigorous phenomenologically-based method' (1996: 384). Varela wrote: '...science proceeds because of its pragmatic link to the phenomenal world; indeed, its validation is derived from the efficacy of this link'.

6 These features subsequently have been elaborated in many works. For an updated review of neuro-phenomenology since Varela's time, see Gallagher and Zahavi 2012.

7 To counter the traditional viewpoint, Varela became editor in the 1990s (along with Jonathon Shear) of the *Journal for Consciousness Studies*, an arena for 'The view from within'. For an expanded view of Francisco Varela's contribution to development of a method for the study of consciousness, see Petitmengin 2009.

8 Varela also elaborated on a theory of *enaction* with his colleague, Evan Thompson (2007). Psychologist Jerome Bruner first defined the word 'enaction' (Bruner 1966). For Bruner, enaction is a way of organizing knowledge (chiefly iconic or symbolic) and of interacting with the world. Maturana and Varela defined it differently, rendering the term synonymous

with interaction and inter-subjectivity in the dynamics of living. Enaction connotes the dynamical exchange between body systems and the environment (Di Paolo, Rohde, and De Jaegher 2010). Enaction is addressed more fully in Chapter 5.

9   Many of Varela's ideas resonate with those of philosopher and Somatics (Feldenkrais) practitioner Thomas Hanna. Hanna advocated for somatology, the science of the human narrative (Hanna 1973). Among the array of pragmatic body and movement-based practices considered 'privileged mediators of change' within this science (Varela and Shear 1999: 4).

10   Debate within cognitive neuroscience remains strongly resistant to the validity of studying conscious experience. Daniel Dennett, for example, states that the phenomenological approach to brain science is '[a] discipline with no methods, no data, no results, no future, no promise…' (Dennett 2001, quoted in Gallagher and Zahavi 2012: 15).

11   Experience was considered the 'hard problem' of cognitive science – how to capture and explain it (Chalmers 1995; 1999). The neuro-phenomenological method was Varela's answer to addressing the hard problem (Varela 1996).

Chapter 5

Enaction

Overview

Since the late nineteenth century, scientists classified kinesthesia as a sensory modality delimiting body position and motion. Albeit reductionist, this perspective was critical to the development of western medical diagnosis. For performing artists, kinesthesia is integral to embodied experience and aesthetic expression – bodily consciousness that enables empathic attunement. While the arts and sciences still seek compatibility on the subject of kinesthesia, embodied cognitive science offers another theory: *enaction*. Fraught with capacity, capability and potential, humans enact experience. In enaction theory, kinesthesia is linked to five core interdigitated values – autonomy, sense-making, embodiment, emergence and experience. In the 1970s, scientists Humberto Maturana, Francisco Varela and later, Evan Thompson, spearheaded the theory of *enaction* to explain the gestalt of experience. Today, enaction theory continues to ripple through a number of scholarly circles (Malkemus 2012). This chapter provides a brief overview of kinesthesia, shifting from a positivist science perspective to an enactive one. The update helps dancers consider the utility of enaction theory as a synthetic approach to studying embodied cognition in dancemaking.

Focusing in…

- How does contemporary neuroscience define kinesthesia?
- Does the scientific perspective have utility for dance training?
- Describe the *meta*-qualities of kinesthesia and their relevance to dance training.
- Describe the theory of *enaction* and elaborate on its core values.
- What principles and concepts complement these values in dance and Somatics?
- What does dance offer that advances *enaction* theory?

Experiential prelude

Observe your body in standing. Notice all the sensations you feel and get a baseline reading on what it feels like to stand up. Pay particular attention to the sensations you feel in your legs, how you are sensing your weight and your ground contact. Now, sit down and place your left palm on your left knee. Become aware of the many kinesthetic and proprioceptive sensations coming from your hand-to-knee contact. What basic vitality is under your hand? What lets you know you are alive? Describe all the sensations you feel – temperature, shape, density etc. Without mentally directing yourself to move in any particular way, note the directions that manifest from your point of contact. In what directions are these energetic *vectors* going? How far from your hand can you extend this sense from your point of contact – to the floor, below the floor, back to your hip and trunk? Notice how kinesthesia is both the perception of sensation and of movement. Notice the reflexivity of touch – the sense of your hand touching your knee and your knee touching your hand. Bring your awareness to that side of your body making contact with your hand, the floor and the chair. Notice the spread of connection between the point of contact and other parts of the body. Now, stand again and compare the difference between your two sides. What differences exist now on your left side? Stand on each leg separately. Which leg provides greater ease of support and readiness to move? Try taking one step forward. Which leg affords greater ease and stability in accepting your weight?

Introduction

The topic of kinesthesia has fascinated and confounded philosophers, scientists and artists across the ages. The term came into use among late nineteenth- and early twentieth-century neuroscientists. The etymological root of the word *kinesthesia* derives from the Greek root *kinein* (to move) and *esthesia* (feeling or perception). The suffixes *aesthesis* and *aisthesis* relate movement to pleasure and beauty. These etymological roots suggest that the founders of modern science might have understood something about the phenomenological and aesthetic dimensions of this sensory endowment (Paterson 2012).[1]

In dance, honing the kinesthetic sense is a vital part of praxis and performance (Clarke, Cramer and Müller 2010; Martin 1939). Cultivating sensitivity, sense-ability and response-ability are vital to 'forming relationships between the interior self and others' (van Manen 2007: 12). For dance scholars, the word kinesthesia ramified over the last few decades to encompass a broad range of subjectively perceived qualities, including movement dynamics, empathy and action observation (Foster 2011; Reynolds and Reason 2012), body-based consciousness (Sheets-Johnstone 2009a; 2009b; Berthoz 2000; Morris 2010; Paterson 2012) and agency (Noland 2009; Freeman 2008).

During this time, cognitive scientists also began to view kinesthesia within the holism of perception and action. Kinesthesia *enacts*; it brings forth experience through the unity of sensing, perceiving and moving. Scientist Humberto Maturana, his protégé Francisco Varela and later, philosopher Evan Thompson, advanced a theory of enaction, from the 1970s to the turn of the twenty-first century (Thompson 2007). Enaction is comprised of five interdigitated phenomena: autonomy, embodiment, sense-making, emergence and experience. Together, these phenomena form a matrix for understanding cognition-as-action (Gapenne 2010). This chapter refreshes the perspectives on kinesthesia within cognitive neuroscience first with an aim toward resolving polarized views of the subject. Second, the chapter alludes to the relevancy of enaction theory in discussions on kinesthesia within dance.

Kinesthesia: positivist roots

Kinesthesia has been a source of fascination from the ancient Greeks onward.[2] In the late nineteenth and early twentieth centuries, the topic came into focus with the rise in modern western neuroscience. Scientists throughout Europe began to classify the senses into separate categories. In England, neuroscientist Sir Charles Bell referred to *'muscle sense'* (Bell 1826) to describe the feeling state of *muscular* movement. Henry Charlton Bastian (1880) advocated using the term *kinesthesia* instead, based on the fact that additional afferent feedback (tendons, joints and skin) gave rise to these sensations (Boring 1942: 525). British father of neuroscience, Sir Charles Sherrington, coined the term *proprioception*, from the Latin *proprius* (one's own), and *percipere*, to perceive (Mosby 2009: 1285). By 1906, *proprioception* replaced kinesthesia as the term of choice for the feeling state of muscles and related tissues associated with bodily positions and movements.

Kinesthesia and proprioception are interrelated sensory phenomena. Both terms are used interchangeably, although discrepancies exist, and distinctions in the scientific literature are hard to find with any degree of consistency (Stillman 2002; Proske 2006). Proprioception generally refers more to localized muscular sensations of the body (Stillman 2002). Kinesthesia locates the body in space and is represented as two sensations: a static sense of spatial location (position) (Barrack and Skinner 1990) and a dynamic sense (moving) (Warner et al. 1996; Gardner and Martin 2000). Static position sense refers to sensory information issuing from stationary orientation of the body, and the relationship of its parts; dynamic sense incorporates neuromuscular and mechanical feedback about the rate, amplitude, direction and force of movement (Ergan and Ulkar 2008).

Motor control science recognizes kinesthesia and proprioception as vital neuromuscular processes underlying body orientation, postural control and balance across the life span (Horak 2006). More fundamentally, kinesthesia and proprioception monitor complex sensations related to maintaining balance and the general facility of moving in gravity (Sheets-Johnstone 2011b: 217). These senses find their origins deep in evolutionary history of 'sentience' and 'surface recognition sensitivity' (Sheets-Johnstone 2011b: 460, 464 – after Curtis and Barnes 1989).

Kinesthetic and proprioceptive data derive from *afferent nerve signals*, located in numerous end organs throughout the body. These end organs are located in muscles, tendons, joints, ligaments, fascia and other tissues of the skeletal, muscle and organ systems. These small sensory nerve endings are *mechanotransducers*, that is, they fire when they are mechanically deformed through touch and movement. Afferent nerve endings activate in response to stretch, pressure, velocity and other information specific to experiencing stillness and movement. Through an act of neurological transduction, afferent neural signals ascend through the spinal cord to the brain where neural processing renders a sense of muscular effort, bodily position and joint motion. Current views support three levels of processing: first-level processing is the non-conscious sensory processing related to the state of bodily condition and position; second-level processing is (sub)cortical, designed to guide and refine action; and third-level processing is conscious kinesthetic awareness related to the complex processing of empathy and other emotions (Gallese and Sinigaglia 2011). Details on these higher levels of neurological processing remain conjectural (Morris 2010).

The reductionist approach of specifying sensory receptor qualities has proven notoriously difficult to unravel (Gandevia 1996). At the same time, single-system sensory testing remains the clinical standard in western medical diagnosis to this day. Single-system data is vital for injury rehabilitation and therapeutic maintenance of neuro-degenerative declines. Clinical specialists can know the status of an injury by the discrete neural pathways involved and the degree to which sensation is altered or lost. If damage results in diminishing sensation, then objective measures play an important role in stages of recovery. At the same time, sensory testing does not provide us with a 'coherent representation' of the whole moving body (Jola 2010: 216). Sensory signals coming from the body are abundant (or – to use the more scientific term – *redundant*) (Barlow 2001). The human body allegedly has at least five times more sensory- than motor nerves. Fortunately, most of this sensory information is non-conscious. Complex processes of inhibition and integration – from spinal reflex arcs to the cortex – turn raw data into useful information. These processes afford humans the ability to ignore the constant barrage of sensations and simply concentrate on attending to tasks at hand.[3]

Dance science researchers have compared kinesthetic abilities in dancers vs. non-dancers on select outcomes, such as position sense and balance. Results have been surprising and counterintuitive (Batson 2009). While position sense in elite dancers appears more accurate than that of novice dancers (Ramsay and Ridoch 2001; Jola, Davis and Haggard 2011), elite dancers demonstrate no particular advantage over other trained athletes on select measures of balance and performance (Perrin 2002). Further, proprioceptive acuity depends on the type of movement executed (Bronner 2012), degree of dependency on vision (Golomer et al. 1999a; 1999b), previous injury (Leanderson 1996) and cognitive clarity (Krasnow 1994). Some suggest that dancers' inaccuracies in joint position testing might stem from generating inefficient mental images. On the other hand, researchers speculate that while these mental images may be inefficient in producing exact joint angles during testing, they might serve practical functions in executing movement (Jola, Davis and Haggard 2011).

Contemporary neuroscience

Scientists recognized early that the importance of kinesthesia was not just a matter of sensation alone, but was intimately tied up with action (Head and Holmes 1911). Contemporary neuroscience has not consistently advanced a principle of perception-action unity, however.[4] Discoveries over the last century, however, have advanced a more holistic understanding of kinesthetic sensibility. Brain-mapping (imaging) studies have been integral to the scientific understanding. Areas of research include: (1) neuroplasticity – the degree to which the brain changes with use (Bütefisch et al. 2000); (2) body image and body schema as representations of self and action (Gallagher 2005; Gallagher and Schmickling 2010);[5] (3) deafferentation (loss of sensation). These studies show that it is possible to move without kinesthetic sensation. The movement may even appear *normal*. Without sensation, however, an unfathomable amount of mental and visual attention is required to control the simplest of actions (Cole 1995; Cole, Gallagher and McNeil 2002); and (4) the mirror neuron system and empathy. Neuroscientists suggest that the mirror neuron network underlies empathic expression and empowers action (Gallese and Sinigaglia 2011). Observing movement, for example, evokes a sympathetic response of similar muscles and/or motor neuron pathways (e.g., Decety et al. 2002; Fadiga et al. 1995). To 'perceive' is to feel and to feel is to 'do'.

Dancers resonate with mirror neuron theory because kinesthetic empathy is a palpable phenomenon.[6] In dancemaking, kinesthesia is a sense-able system with two-way perception capability, active and reflexive. When we perceive other dancers moving, we feel our own experience (Sklar 1994). Movement readily is felt, empathized with, mimicked, intuited and re-enacted, even when we merely observe another's actions (Gallese 2006; Freedberg and Gallese 2007). Studies on kinesthetic empathy and action observation on watching dance have been compelling. Watching dance evokes 'sympathetic kinaesthesia' (Stevens et al. 2003: 320). Portions of the mirror neuron system of the brain activate preferentially when either dancers watch other dancers (Calvo-Merino et al. 2005; 2008), or when audiences watch dance (Jola, Ehrenberg and Reynolds 2012).

Kinesthesia and movement – a phenomenological gestalt

Despite the extensive research on the mirror neuron system, scientists critique these discoveries as another effort to localize brain functions (e.g., Hicock 2009). Dance phenomenologists, too, take scientists to task. *Movement*, not specialized visuo-motor neurons in the mirror neuron system, is the fundamental baseline of empathic communication (Sheets-Johnstone 2012b). Movement is not a neural construct, but an experience that gives rise to a range of dynamics and impressions (Sheets-Johnstone 2012b; 2011a), deepening all relationships in growth and development.

This kinesthesia-as-movement system 'is constitutive of, not tangential to, the process of individuation' (Noland 2009: 10). Life span development hinges on making sense of experience through the feeling states of movement (Freyd 1983; Thelen and Smith 1994; Bainbridge Cohen 1993; Behnke 2008). Developmental scientists considered kinesthesia fundamental to babies' emotional growth and social attachment (Schore 1994). Human resonance and responsiveness begins in utero through the integrated experience of movement, touch and kinesthesia.[6] Movement sensations are 'connection-seeking and relation-making' (Stafford 2011: 65). These are the vital 'precursors of empathy', underscoring developmental attachment and attunement (Berrol 2006: 308), the underpinnings of inter-subjectivity and social communication (Schore 1994).

Cognitive science and enaction

Enter the *theory of enaction*. Enaction was designed to help bridge the gap between mind and experience. Biologist Humberto Maturana and his protégé Francisco Varela adopted the term *enaction* in the late 1970s as part of a constructivist concept of embodied cognition (Stewart, Gapenne and Di Paolo 2010).[7] Enaction is a unified, embodied form of perception and action (Thompson 2007). Enacting brings forth reality. The authors proposed the term enaction 'to emphasize the growing conviction that cognition is not the representation of a pregiven world by a pregiven mind but is rather the enactment of a world and a mind on the basis of a history of the variety of actions that a being in the world performs' (Varela, Thompson and Rosch 1991: 9).

Enactivists do not view the brain as the primary controller of thought, feeling and action (Fuchs 2011; Varela, Thompson and Rosch 1991). Rather, cognition is for action (Wilson 2002). Scientist Alva Noë states: 'Experience is not something we have but something we *do* and that we do as a consequence of relating to our environment. Without a world, there would be no perception. As for consciousness, we enact it, with the world's help, in our dynamic living activities. It is not something that happens to us' (Noë 2009: 64). Enaction is rooted in biological movement – embodied and dynamical – constantly exchanging information with the environment (Di Paolo, Rohde and De Jaegher 2010).

Enaction embraces five core values issuing from the coupling of brain, body and world: 'autonomy, embodiment, sense-making, emergence and experience' (DiPaolo, Rohde and De Jaegher 2010: 33, 37).[8] Enaction thrives as living, situated engagement (Varela1999; Fuchs 2011; Thompson and Varela 2001; Thompson 2007; Wilson and Foglia 2011). Our moving eyes are located in a moving head on a moving body in a moving world (Gibson 1979).

'Natural cognitive systems…participate in the generation of meaning through their bodies and action often engaging in *transformational*…not merely *informational* interactions' (Di Paolo, Rohde and De Jaegher 2010: 39 – italics Batson's). These interactions give rise to flexible and adaptive dynamics, 'styles of relating' (Schmidt 2011: 33). They underscore self-awareness, skill and social interaction (Di Paolo, Rohde and De Jaegher 2010; Lewis and Todd 2007). As Schmidt (2011) notes: 'By bringing my body into the movie theatre, I have brought in a locus for multiple, overlapping and cross-modal styles of perceptual relationship. I do have the ability to manoeuvre within these relationships, but I cannot shut them off' (2011: 40).

Implications for dancemakers

Dance scholars are divided on the usefulness of enaction theory in explaining the kinesthetic underpinnings of dance. Proponents support the theory as a means of 're-languaging' dance experience (Warburton 2011: 67). The model of enaction encompasses three intertwined modes of bodily action that resonate with dance experience: 'self-regulation (somatic realm), sensorimotor coupling (kinesthetic realm) and intersubjective interaction (mimetic, simulating realm)' (Warburton 2011: 69).

At the same time, critics state that enaction theory 'falls short of doing justice to the spatiotemporal-energetic qualitative dynamics of affect and movement and falls short equally of realizing their dynamically congruent relationship…By focusing mainly on sense-making bodies, enaction theory tends toward reducing movement dynamics to faculties or actions, rather than primal relationships. Our strength of connection, communication and relationship in the world lies in our experience *as animate beings* not in our brain' (Sheets-Johnstone 2011b: 455).[9] Dancemakers can continue to test the utility of enaction as they thicken their descriptions of dance experience.

Explorations for this chapter appear in Appendix II.

References

Barlow, H. (2001), 'Redundancy reduction revisited', *Network: Computation in Neural Systems*, 12: 3, pp. 241–53.

Barrack, R. and Skinner, H. (1990), 'The sensory function of knee ligaments', *Knee Ligaments: Structure, Function, Injury and Repair*, New York, NY: Raven, pp. 95–114.

Batson, G. (2009), 'The somatic practice of intentional rest in dance education – preliminary steps towards a method of study', *Journal of Dance and Somatic Practices*, 1: 2, pp. 177–97.

Behnke, E. (2008), 'Interkinesthetic affectivity: A phenomenological approach', *Continental Philosophy Review*, 41: 2, pp. 143–61.

Bell, C. (1826), 'On the nervous circle which connects the voluntary muscles with the brain', *Philosophical Transactions of the Royal Society of London*, 116: 1/3, pp. 163–73.

Berrol, C.F. (2006), 'Neuroscience meets dance/movement therapy: Mirror neurons, the therapeutic process and empathy', *The Arts in Psychotherapy*, 33: 4, pp. 302–15.

Berthoz, A. (2000), *The Brain's Sense of Movement*, Cambridge, MA: Harvard University Press.

Boring, E. (1942), *Sensation and Perception in the History of Experimental Psychology*, New York, NY: Appleton-Century.

Bronner, S. (2012), 'Differences in segmental coordination and postural control in a multi-joint dance movement: développé arabesque', *Journal of Dance Medicine and Science*, 16: 1, pp. 26–35.

Bruner, J. (1962), *The Process of Education*, Cambridge, MA: Harvard University Press.

——— (1966), *Toward a Theory of Instruction*, Cambridge, MA: Belknap Press of Harvard University Press.

Bütefisch, C.M., Davis, B.C., Wise, S.P. et al. (2000), 'Mechanisms of use-dependent plasticity in the human motor cortex', *Proceeds of the National Academy of Science*, 97: 2, pp. 3661–65.

Calvo-Merino, B., Glaser, D.E., Passingham, R.E. and Haggard, P. (2005), 'Action observation and acquired motor skills: An fMRI study with expert dancers', *Cerebral Cortex*, 15: 8, pp. 1243–49.

Calvo-Merino, B., Jola, C., Glaser, D.E. and Haggard, P. (2008), 'Towards a sensorimotor aesthetics of performing art', *Consciousness and Cognition*, 17, pp. 911–22.

Clarke, G., Cramer, F. and Müller, G. (2010), 'Minding motion' in I. Diehl and F. Lampert (eds.), *Dance Techniques 2010*, Leipzig: Henschel Verlag, pp. 199–229.

Cohen, B.B. (1993), *Sensing, Feeling, and Action: The Experiential Anatomy of Body-Mind Centering*, Northampton, MA: Contact Editions.

Cole, J. (1995), *Pride and a Daily Marathon*, Cambridge, MA: MIT Press.

Cole, J., Gallagher, S. and McNeill, D. (2002), 'Gesture following deafferentation: A phenomenologically informed experimental study', *Phenomenology and the Cognitive Sciences*, 1: 1, pp. 49–67.

Cole, J. and Montero, B. (2007), 'Affective proprioception', *Janus Head*, 9: 2, pp. 299–317.

Decety, J., Chaminade, T., Grèzes, J. and Meltzoff, A. (2002), 'A PET exploration of the neural mechanisms involved in reciprocal imitation', *NeuroImage*, 15: 1, pp. 265–72.

Di Paolo, E., Rohde, M. and De Jaegher, H. (2010), 'Horizons for the enactive mind: Values, social interaction, and play' in J. Stewart, O. Gapenne and E. Di Paolo (eds.), *Enaction: Towards a New Paradigm for Cognitive Science*, Cambridge, MA: MIT Press, pp. 33–88.

Ergen, E. and Ulkar, B. (2008), 'Proprioception and ankle injuries in soccer', *Clinics in Sports Medicine*, 27: 1, pp. 195–217.

Fadiga, L., Fogassi, L., Pavesi, G. and Rizzolatti, G. (1995), 'Motor facilitation during action observation: A magnetic stimulation study', *Journal of Neurophysiology*, 73: 6, pp. 2608–11.

Foster, S. (2011), *Choreographing Empathy: Kinesthesia in Performance*, London/New York: Routledge.

Freedberg, D. and Gallese, V. (2007), 'Motion, emotion and empathy in esthetic experience, *Trends in the Cognitive Sciences*, 11: 5, pp. 197–203.

Freeman, W. (2008), 'Perception of time and causation through the kinesthesia of intentional action', *Integrative Psychological and Behavioral Science*, 42: 2, pp. 137–43.

Freyd, J. (1983), 'Representing the dynamics of a static form', *Memory and Cognition*, 11: 4, pp. 342–46.

Fuchs, T. (2011), 'The brain – A mediating organ', *Journal of Consciousness Studies*, 18: 7–8, pp. 196–221.

Gallagher, S. (2005), *How the Body Shapes the Mind*, Oxford: Oxford University Press.

Gallagher, S. and Schmicking, D. (2010), *Handbook of Phenomenology and Cognitive Science*, New York, NY: Springer.

Gallese, V. (2006), 'Mirror neurons and intentional attunement', *Journal of the American Psychoanalytic Association*, 54: 1, pp. 47–57.

Gallese, V. and Sinigaglia, C. (2011), 'What is so special about embodied simulation?', *Trends in the Cognitive Sciences*, 15: 11, pp. 512–19.

Gandevia, S.G. (1996), 'Kinesthesia: Roles for afferent signals and motor commands', *Comprehensive Physiology*, Supplement 29, http://onlinelibrary.wiley.com/doi/10.1002/cphy.cp120104/full. Accessed 24 September 2013.

Gapenne, O. (2010), 'Kinesthesia and the construction of perceptual objects' in J. Stewart, O. Gapenne and E.A. Di Paolo (eds.), *Enaction: Toward a New Paradigm for Cognitive Science*, London: MIT Press, pp. 183–218.

Gardner, E. and Martin, J. (2000), 'Coding of sensory information', *Principles of Neural Science*, 4, pp. 411–29.

Gibson, J. (1979), *The Ecological Approach to Visual Perception*, Boston: Houghton Mifflin.

Golomer, E., Dupui, P., Séréni, P. and Monod, H. (1999a), 'The contribution of vision in dynamic spontaneous sways of male classical dancers according to student or professional level', *Journal of Physiology of Paris*, 93: 3, pp. 233–37.

Golomer, E., Crémieux, J., Dupui, P., Isableu, B. and Ohlmann, T. (1999b), 'Visual contribution to self-induced body sway frequencies and visual perception of male professional dancers', *Neuroscience Letters*, 267: 3, pp. 189–92.

Head, H. and Holmes, G. (1911), 'Sensory disturbances from cerebral lesions', *Brain*, 34: 2–3, pp. 102–254.

Hickok, G. (2009), 'Eight problems for the mirror neuron theory of action understanding in monkeys and humans', *Journal of Cognitive Neuroscience*, 21: 7, pp. 1229–43.

Horak, F. (2006), 'Postural orientation and equilibrium: What do we need to know about neural control of balance to prevent falls?', *Age Ageing*, 35: 2, pp. :ii7–ii11.

Jola, C. (2010), 'Research and choreography' in B. Bläsing, M. Puttke and T. Schack (eds.), *The Neurocognition of Dance: Mind, Movement and Motor Skills*, New York, NY: Psychology Press.

Jola, C., Davis, A. and Haggard, P. (2011), 'Proprioceptive integration and body representation: Insights into dancers' expertise', *Experimental Brain Research*, 213: 2–3, pp. 257–65.

Jola, C., Ehrenberg, S. and Reynolds, D. (2012), 'The experience of watching dance: Phenomenological-neuroscience duets', *Phenomenology and the Cognitive Sciences*, 11: 1, pp. 17–37.

Krasnow, D. (1994), 'Performance, movement and kinesthesia', *Impulse*, 2, pp. 16–23.

Leanderson, J., Eriksson, E., Nilsson, C. and Wykman, A. (1996), 'Proprioception in classical ballet dancers. A prospective study of the influence of an ankle sprain on proprioception in the ankle joint', *American Journal of Sports Medicine*, 24: 3, pp. 370–74.

Lewis, M.D. and Todd, R. (2007), 'The self-regulating brain: Cortical-subcortical feedback and the development of intelligent action', *Cognitive Development*, 22, pp. 406–30.

Malkemus, S.A. (2012), 'Toward a general theory of enaction: Biological, transpersonal, and phenomenological dimensions', *The Journal of Transpersonal Psychology*, 44: 2, pp. 201–23.

Martin, J. (1939/1965), *Introduction to the Dance*, republication of 1939 edn, New York, NY: Dance Horizons.

Maturana, H. and Varela, F. (1992), *The Tree of Knowledge: The Biological Roots of Human Understanding* (rev. edn), Boston, MA: Shambala.

Morris, D. (2010), 'Empirical and phenomenological studies of embodied cognition', *Handbook of Phenomenology and Cognitive Science*, Netherlands: Springer, pp. 235–52.

Mosby Staff (2009), *Mosby's Medical Dictionary*, 8th edn, New York, NY: Elsevier.

Noë, A. (2009), *Out of Our Heads: Why You Are Not Your Brain, and Other Lessons From the Biology of Consciousness*, New York, NY: Hill and Wang.

Noland, C. (2009), *Agency and Embodiment: Performing Gestures/Producing Culture*, Cambridge, MA: Harvard University Press.

Paterson, M. (2012), 'Movement for movement's sake? On the relationship between kinesthesia and aesthetics', *Essays in Philosophy*, 13: 2, pp. 471–97.

Perrin, P., Deviterne, D., Hugel, F. and Perrot, C. (2002), 'Judo, better than dance, develops sensorimotor adaptabilities involved in balance control', *Gait and Posture*, 15: 2, pp. 187–94.

Proske, U. (2006), 'Kinesthesia: The role of muscle receptors', *Muscle Nerve*, 34: 5, pp. 545–58.

Ramsay, J. and Riddoch, M. (2001), 'Position-matching in the upper limb: Professional ballet dancers perform with outstanding accuracy', *Clinical Rehabilitation*, 15: 3, pp. 324–30.

Reynolds, D. and Reason, M. (eds.) (2012), *Kinesthetic Empathy in Creative and Cultural Practices*, Bristol/Chicago: Intellect Books.

Schmidt, L. (2011), 'Sound matters: Towards an enactive approach to hearing media', *The Soundtrack*, 4: 1, pp. 33–42.

Schore, A.N. (1994), *Affect Regulation and the Origin of the Self: The Neurobiology of Emotional Development*, Mahwah, NJ: Erlbaum.

Sheets-Johnstone, M. (2009a), *The Corporeal Turn: An Interdisciplinary Reader*, Charlottesville, VA: Imprint Academic.

Sheets-Johnstone, M. (2009b), 'Animation: The fundamental, essential, and properly descriptive concept', *Continental Philosophy Review*, 42: 3, pp. 375–400.

Sheets-Johnstone, M. (2011a), 'From movement to dance', *Phenomenology and the Cognitive Sciences*, 11: 1, pp. 39–57.

Sheets-Johnstone, M. (2011b), *The Primacy of Movement*, expanded 2nd edn, Philadelphia, PA: John Benjamin's Publishing Company.

Sheets-Johnstone, M. (2012a), 'Fundamental and inherently interrelated aspects of animation' in A. Foolen, U.M Ludtke, T.P. Racine and J. Zlatev (eds.), *Moving Ourselves, Moving Others: Motion and Emotion in Intersubjectivity, Consciousness and Language*, Philadelphia, PA: John Benjamin's Publishing Company, pp. 29–56.

Sheets-Johnstone, M. (2012b), 'Movement and mirror neurons: A choice and challenging conversation', *Phenomenology and the Cognitive Sciences*, 11: 3, pp. 385–401.

Shusterman, R. (2004), 'Somaesthetics and education: Exploring the terrain' in L. Bresler (ed.), *Knowing Bodies, Moving Minds: Towards an Embodied Teaching and Learning*, Dordrecht: Kluwer, pp. 51–60.

Sklar, D. (1994), 'Can bodylore be brought to its senses?', *The Journal of American Folklore*, 107: 423, pp. 9–22.

Stafford, B. (ed.) (2011), *A Field Guide to a New Meta-Field: Bridging the Humanities-Neurosciences Divide*, Chicago, IL: University of Chicago Press.

Stillman, B. (2002), 'Making Sense of Proprioception: The meaning of proprioception, kinaesthesia and related terms', *Physiotherapy*, 88: 11, pp. 667–76.

Stevens, C., Malloch, S., McKechnie, S. and, & Steven, N. (2003), 'Choreographic cognition: The time-course and phenomenology of creating a dance', *Pragmatics & Cognition*, 11: 2, pp. 297–326.

Stewart, J. (2010), 'Foundational issues in enaction as a paradigm for cognitive science: From the origin of life to consciousness and writing', in J. Stewart, O. Gapenne, E. Di Paolo (eds.), *Enaction: Toward a New Paradigm for Cognitive Science*, London: MIT Press.

Thelen, E. and Smith, L. (1996), *A Dynamic Systems Approach to the Development of Cognition and Action*, Cambridge, MA: MIT press.

Thompson, E. and Varela, F. (2001), 'Radical embodiment: Neural dynamics and consciousnesses', *Trends in the Cognitive Sciences*, 5: 10, pp. 418–25.

Thompson, E. (2007), *Mind in Life: Biology, Phenomenology, and the Sciences of Mind*, Cambridge, MA: Belknap Press of Harvard University Press.

van Manen, M. (2007), 'Phenomenology of practice', *Phenomenology & Practice*, 1: 1, pp. 11–30.

Varela, F.J. (1999), 'The specious present: A neurophenomenology of time consciousness' in J. Petito, F. Varela, B. Pachoud and J-M Roy (eds.), *Naturalizing Phenomenology: Issues in Contemporary Phenomenology and Cognitive Science*, Stanford, CA: Stanford University Press, pp. 266–314.

Varela, F., Thompson, E. and Rosch, E. (1991), *The Embodied Mind: Cognitive Science and Human Experience*, Cambridge, MA: MIT Press.

Warburton, E. (2011), 'Of meanings and movements: Re-languaging embodiment in dance phenomenology and cognition', *Dance Research Journal*, 43: 2, pp. 65–83.

Warner, J., Lephart, S. and Fu, F. (1996), 'Role of proprioception in pathoetiology of shoulder instability', *Clinical Orthopaedics and Related Research*, 330, pp. 35–39.

Wilson, M. (2002), 'Six views of embodied cognition', *Psychonomic Bulletin and Review*, 9, pp. 625–636.

Wilson, R. and Foglia, L. (2011), 'Embodied cognition', *Stanford Encyclopedia of Philosophy*, http://plato.stanford.edu/entries/embodied-cognition/. Accessed 15 January 2013.

Notes

1   While kinesthesia is intimately associated with aesthetic evaluation and judgment within dance, this chapter does not cover this aspect. Rather, the point here is to advance a neuro-phenomenological perspective on kinesthesia in its capacity to enact experience. For a review of kinesthesia emphasizing aesthetic evaluation, see Paterson 2012; 2006; Cole and Montero 2007; Foster 2011; choreographing empathy, and other sources. The chapter also will not cover kinesthetic empathy. Readers are directed to Reynolds and Reason 2012.

2   For fuller elaboration on the historical background of kinesthesia and the related term proprioception, see Paterson 2012 and Foster 2011, fully cited in the References.

3   Sheets-Johnstone argues that movement is not 'sensational' (2009: 30; 2012a: 30). Kinesthesia is an 'experience of one's own movement…not a matter of sensations but of dynamics' (Sheets-Johnstone 2009a: 225). Sensations are '*temporally punctual…*[and]…*spatially pointillist*' (Sheets-Johnstone 2011b: 511).

4   Critics state that neuroscientists neglect to evaluate the role of kinesthesia in experience and movement. Dance phenomenologist Maxine Sheets-Johnstone argues that, '[t]he kinesthetic moving body should be at the forefront rather than the hind end of scientific investigations' (Sheets-Johnstone 2011a: 147). Sheets-Johnstone reviewed eight contemporary neuroscience texts, each giving only perfunctory acknowledgments to proprioception as important in 'position' and 'information…without any reference to movement and its inherent spatio-temporal-energic dynamics' (Sheets-Johnstone 2011a: 147–48). Additionally, she critiques

those delimiting kinesthesia to a minor role in voluntary movement (position sense) or element within brain schema of self (Sheets-Johnstone 2011a; 2011b; 2009a).

5   These discoveries come as no surprise to dance or somatic praxis. Cultivating kinesthetic sensibility is a shared value, although means and ends may differ. Humans constantly are 'making a body' in encountering gravity, people and context (Behnke 1997: 186) that is representational and experiential (Schusterman, in Bresler 2004: 53).

6   Dance scholar John Martin wrote as early as 1936: 'When we see a human body moving, we see movement which is potentially producible by a human body and therefore by our own; through kinesthetic sympathy we actually reproduce it vicariously in our present muscular experience and awaken such associational connotations as might have been ours if the original movement had been of our own making. The irreducible minimum of equipment demanded of a spectator, therefore, is a kinesthetic sense in working condition' (Martin 1936: 117).

7   Again, Sheets-Johnstone gives primacy to animation and movement as underlying growth and development (2009a; 2009b; 2011a; 2011b).

8   The basic concepts of enaction are elaborated in *The Tree of Knowledge* (Varela and Maturana 1992). Varela later embellished this theory with his colleague, philosopher Evan Thompson (Thompson and Varela 2001). Interestingly, the core attributes of enaction parallel those values embedded in the somatic education and praxis, although not explicitly stated within the somatic literature as such.

9   For a critique of enaction theory, see Chapter 13 'Animation' in M. Sheets-Johnstone (2011), *The Primacy of Movement*, expanded 2nd edn.

Chapter 6

Attention and Effort

We have no sensation of the inner workings of the central nervous system…as the sensation of effort is not a measure of the work done but an indicator of the degree and quality of organization producing the effort…Thus the sensation of no-effort in action is present not at no-work but at correctly co-ordinated work.

(Moshe Feldenkrais 1964: 79, 84)

The body is made up of what it learns to discern….

(Bar-On Cohen 2006: 77)

A glimpse of the next four chapters

Attention is the ability to remain focused on relevant information in the presence of distractions. In dancemaking, focused attention to augmented states of embodiment is the essence of movement practice. Attention is tethered to moment-to-moment changes within bodily- and contextual dynamics. Functioning as a kind *attunement*, attention is critical to artistic communication and performance. This chapter is one of four companion chapters opening discussion on the topic of training attention within dance. First, we offer a primer on attention training derived from cognitive and sports psychology. Central to the discussion is the relationship between mental and physical effort in honing physical skill. While this complex relationship is not well understood, it nonetheless figures into pedagogical design. Science supports the use of *mental* protocols for training attention, a popular example being mindfulness training. Somatic learning, on the other hand, prefaces embodied movement practices wherein attending to bodily sensations[1] coordinates mind and body. While somatic learning has benefited dancers in many ways, the topic of attention rarely has taken center stage in discussions on performance enhancement.

Focusing in…

- What is attention? What is meant by *control* of attention?
- What are different *styles* of attention?
- Describe the state of effortlessness? How can it be achieved?
- What current models of attention training enhance dance technique and performance?

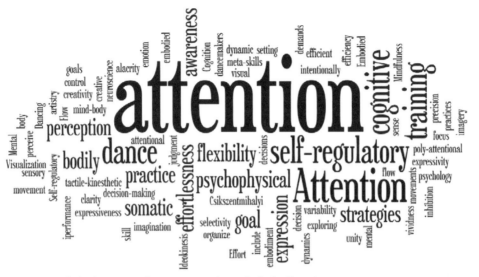

Figure 6.1: *Word Cloud:* Foregrounding attention within embodied self-regulatory processes.

Experiential prelude

In ancient Sanskrit, the word for attention is *dhyana*, meaning 'the long, pure look' (Sewell 1999: 100). This phrase implies a long time frame of unhindered, meditative focus. Right now, consciously and deliberately order yourself to '*pay attention*' to reading this material. What change in your bodily attitude do you experience? Do you notice a quickening, a narrowing and a tightening of body tonus as you do this? Where? Now, forget that directive. Relax your attention and breathe for a minute or so, letting go of focusing on anything particular. Then…

1. Focus on your knee as you are sitting there. Notice the quality and the duration of your focus. In attending, what kinesthetic sensations are you aware of? How readily do you feel the urge to shift your attention to something else?
2. Focus on the kinesthetic sensations of your knee as you slowly extend it. How does paying attention to this action affect your focus – its quality, scope, feeling of effort etc.?
3. Extend your knee as *effortlessly* as possible. What shift in you takes place to go from merely performing the function to extending your knee effortlessly?
4. Extend your focus to encompass your environment as you extend your knee. Now, how is your attention affected? What effect does the expanded field of attention have on your sense of effortlessness?

5. Can you focus on several things at once? Extending your knee while writing down your perceptions at the same time?
6. Stand up. Compare both knees as you stand and remain standing. Which knee feels more *effortless*? What synonyms would you add to a sense of effortlessness?
7. Pick up a material object that weighs about 5 pounds, such as a large stone. Notice the effort it takes to lift and hold it. Your head weighs approximately 25 pounds. Which feels heavier, the object or your head? How do you account for the difference? What would need to change in your perception or coordination to lift the material object effortlessly?

As you are reading this chapter, think about the many factors that imprint on your habits of attention – biological, sociocultural, technological and training. How do these factors influence your style of attending, your flexibility in switching tasks and the endurance of your focus? How would you describe your habits as you attend to a common everyday task, such as making pasta for dinner? For dancers, think of an example of how you attend when you are learning new dance moves. Do you have a habitual manner and style of attending in learning dance? How would you go about changing it, if you wanted to?

Track how your attention fluctuates over a typical day and record your observations in a journal. Start to build a personal vocabulary to describe your habits of attending.

The state of things

Among the many cognitive faculties, attention is vital to developing safe, effective and aesthetic dancing (Taylor 2011; Grove, Stevens and McKechnie 2005; Moffitt 2012). For psychologists, attention is a multidimensional construct critical to self-regulatory control (Hossner and Wenderoth 2009; Bargh and Chartrand 1999). A thorough grasp of the subject requires integrating theories from cognitive neuroscience, phenomenology, dynamic systems theory, exercise and sports science, eco-psychology, cultural studies, anthropology and more (Bruya 2010). At the same time, the lack of domain- and activity-specific definitions for attention remains a major obstacle to advancing theory (Nakamura and Csikszentmihalyi 2002; Simonton 2007). Further, capturing the scope of attention in research models remains challenging (Mole 2013; Gruzka, Matthews and Szymura 2010).

Despite theoretical lags, however, numerous training methods are now available to the lay public, offering a number of ways to improve the skills of attention. These methods largely address cognitive deficits or declines, and aim toward developing a sense of control.[2] Justifiably, the arts (including dance) are considered effective in training attention (Posner and Patoine 2009). Dance offers multimodal experiences linking cognition to embodied states (Stevens and McKechnie 2005). Dancing stimulates an array of cognitive processes – awareness, perception, attention, imagination, insight, problem-solving, decision-making, judgment, memory and recall. Recent studies point to the positive impact of dance on cognitive processes in child development (Balgeonkar 2010; Ashbury and Rich 2008) and among the elderly (Coubard et al. 2011; Kattenstroth et al. 2010; 2011; 2013; Kim et al. 2011; Ferrufino et al. 2011; Jovancevic et al. 2012; Giguere 2011). Although results from these studies do not generalize to elite performers, dance offers ample opportunity to practice 'higher order' cognitive skills (Moffett 2012: 1).[3]

In dance, attention is embodied and destined toward artistic communication. Dancers harness their attention to creating and honing movement. In this way, attention acts as *sensory* or *perceptual* attunement (Dormashev 2010). Dancers attune to a range of movement dynamics in mastering physical skills. Body and mind are unified in negotiating the changing space, time and effort dynamics. Gaining expertise in dance includes developing flexible and adaptive attentional skills. General skills, for example, include a (supra-normal) ability to avoid distractions that interfere with negotiating complex movement tasks and environments. Simultaneously, dancers must learn to redirect attention toward more optimal conditions. Dancers also develop a multiplicity of *styles* of attention specific to various dance forms or choreographic demands. These styles impact on communication, expression and meaning.

Attention is a cognitive process critical to self-regulatory control. Dancers cope with performance stresses through an array of psychophysical skills, such as managing the amount of information at any one time and lowering anxiety. One vital skill in becoming a dance artist lies in regulating the mental cost of physical effort. This is important in all phases of learning and perfecting movement. Skilled coordination is associated with efficiency, effectiveness and a subjective feeling of effortlessness. Unless effortful expression is deliberately choreographed in a dance, psychophysical expressions of effort are masked in service to the aesthetic of *effortlessness* (Bläsing et al. 2012). How this embodied state of effortlessness arises remains mysterious and under-investigated. How is this 'state' achieved, mentally and physically? From what fields can dance researchers best glean an understanding of attention in dance?

One well-validated model for effortless attention in performance is the *flow* model, developed by social scientist Mihaly Csikszentmihalyi. *Flow* is a state of total immersion and absorption in the task at hand, with a commensurate lowering of the level of anxiety (Csikszentmihalyi 1990).[4] This model of psychophysical effortlessness is well validated for many activities. Dance also is mentioned, although the results of Csikszentmihalyi's interviews with dancers are not reported in full in his seminal book *Flow* (1990).

Somatic learning (Somatics) offers a large body of empirical data on the interrelationship of mental and physical effort. Somatics offers pragmatic 'proof' that attention is not only a mental construct. Somatic educators view attention as a basic *somatic* function, fundamental to the capacity and capability for building relationships to self and others (Gold 1992/93). Somatics incorporates a wide spectrum of practices, from contemplative/meditative practices to outwardly expressive movement ones. In Somatics, learners attend to sensory data coming from their interior states, movement and the environment. Initiates enter into somatic learning by perceiving and attending to bodily sensations. Through this and other embodied processes, body and mind are united in the pursuit of self-regulation (Juhan 1986). Attending to sensory dynamics awakens self-regulatory processes needed to build a sense of embodied autonomy and control – physical, mental and emotional. These skills are needed to bridge between inner states and the outer world. This concept is also echoed within embodied cognitive science (Thompson 2010), albeit with the emphasis on *mind* rather than bodymind (Sheets-Johnstone 2011).

A fundamental value in all somatic practices is cultivating sensory sensitivity (Hanlon-Johnson 2000; 2004). The purpose of sensory sensitivity is not merely to *awaken* the body but to *hone perceptual discrimination and discernment*. Paying attention to sensations of muscular tonus (and other sensations arising from moving-thinking) impacts on coordination. By sensitizing and discriminating among sensory phenomena, one learns to distinguish degrees of physical- and mental effort in honing movement skill.[5] In Somatics, learners attend to sensations for a prolonged period of time in an environment of suspended doing (Batson and Schwartz 2007). This sensory-rich field of attention and rest promotes self-regulatory processes related to motor programming (see Chapter 7 for a fuller discussion on the somatic learning environment).

The topic of attention remains wide open for dance research and praxis integration (deLahunta, Clarke and Barnard 2012). Science, too, lacks a gold standard for measuring attention or a tenable theory on processes or skills of attention that optimize artistic performance (Pickens et al. 2010). A literature search revealed only three articles indirectly related to the phenomenon of mental and physical effort in dancemaking: A quantitative study reporting the effects of mentally practicing choreography on cortical 'fatigue' (Blaser and Hökelman 2009), one review of cortical fatigue (Batson 2013) and one qualitative study reporting dancers' responses to resting intentionally (Batson 2009).

Below is a primer on attention from the perspective of cognitive science: What is attention? What skills are needed? What methods improve its control? The overview synthesizes concepts from cognitive neuroscience and sports science/psychology. We bring forth the somatic learning perspective as empirical support for embodied attention training. In doing so, we return to embodied movement training as the baseline for understanding the intricate relationship between attention, effort and coordination. The aim is to recontextualize somatic learning as a potent agent in developing embodied skills of attention that enhance coordination.

Attention: a primer

Attention is a word that derives from the Latin *attendere*, meaning 'to give heed to', literally 'to stretch toward' (Harper 2001–03). Paying attention is an embodied act. We *stretch* ourselves – reaching out with embodied resonance toward the focal point at hand. When the subject of attention surfaced among western intelligentsia during the late nineteenth and early twentieth centuries, it quickly became incorporated into the dominion of the *mental* and the *mind*, losing its connections to embodiment. In 1890, philosopher William James wrote, 'Everyone knows what attention is. It is the taking possession by the mind, in clear and vivid form, of one out of what seem several simultaneously possible objects or trains of thought. Focalization, concentration of consciousness, are of its essence. It implies withdrawal from some things in order to deal effectively with others, and is a condition which has a real opposite in the confused, dazed, scatterbrained state which in French is called distraction, and Zerstreutheit in German' (James 1890: 403–04). James' 'taking possession by the mind' suggests that we have conscious control (choice) over our cognitive processes of focusing and concentrating. In some ways, James set the stage for a dualist concept of attention. His early concepts gave rise to separating attention into a 'top down' mental state (i.e., a goal-driven or *endogenous* process), and a 'bottom up,' or more stimulus-driven, state (a subliminal or *exogenous* process) (from Muraven et al. 1998).

Today, cognitive scientists define attention as 'a series of mental processes that allow for selectively concentrating on one aspect of the environment while simultaneously ignoring other things' (Anderson 2004: 519). Whether the model for attention comes from information processing, phenomenology or human movement science, the fundamental skill of attention lies in 'learning to negotiate perceptual intrusions' (Kinchia 1980: 215). Attention is critical to staying focused against the enormity and volatility of information. It is also selective, extracting relevant information from any task (Kinchia 1980; von Gaal et al. 2012).

Attention is a topic of great interest to contemporary neuroscientists (Posner and Rothbart 1998; Mangun 2011). Attention lies along the spectrum of consciousness – arousal, awareness, attention, action and reflection (Gurwitsch 1964; Arvidson 2010; Dehaene and Nacchace 2001). It is one of the brain's *executive functions*. Executive functions are evolutionarily advanced functions underlying self-regulation of volitional behavior (Powers 2010; Chan et al. 2008; Carver and Scheier 1981). Perception, attention, goal-setting, problem-solving and many different manifestations of memory (such as procedural and working memory) are among these functions (Pickens et al. 2010; Cabeza and Nyberg 1997; Bauer and Zelazo 2013).

From the vantage point of embodied cognition, attention assumes a phenomenological dimension. Attention is a way of expressing being and becoming in the world, of coupling thinking with world-making (Thompson and Stapleton 2008). Attention is *enactive*; it brings forth attachment and bonding in relationships (Varela, Thompson and Rosch 1991). Further, attention exhibits different manners or 'styles' (Schmidt 2011). Styles are manifestations of ways humans exploit space-time-effort qualities to meet task demands and contexts. The kind of attention needed for talking to a friend on a cell phone in a busy café is very different from that needed for improvising alone outdoors on a rock formation.

Sports psychology describes modes of attention as selective or diffuse (narrow or wide-angle focus), divided or sustained (uni- or multifocal) (Bruya 2010: 221–22; Schmeichel and Baumeister 2010: 31, 236; Gill 2000). Spatial styles of attentional focus also incorporate both the vantage point of the viewer as well as whether the viewer is distanced or engaged in the activity (degree of absorption). Visual attention, for example, might operate in the manner of a spotlight, flashlight or penlight, or like a wide angle- or zoom lens. Spatial styles thus can be narrow and subjective (such as making a cell phone call), narrow and objective (fixing a watch), broad and subjective (dancing in an ensemble) and broad and objective (lost in the wide panorama of a desert) (Fehmi and Robbins 2007).[6]

In summary, attention is not one neural function, state, trait, skill or capability but, rather, a dynamical system (Sarter, Gehring and Kozak 2006). Training attention requires learning and mastering many skills. Among these are selectivity, precision and clarity; flexibility and duration of focus; quickness and agility in shifting; and a full spectrum of dynamic styles. Training also must take into consideration biological and sociocultural characteristics, the impact of technology and the specifics of context and task demands. These, and other factors, impact on styles and habits of attention, as well (Peh, Chow and Davids 2011).

Attention: capacity and control

Four complex neurological processes are essential for attentional control: (1) monitoring the amount of information we attend to (the cognitive 'load') (Paas, Renkel and Sweller 2004); (2) reducing any excessive impulsive or distractive behaviors/emotions (inhibitory control) (Bari and Robbins 2013); (3) calibrating the rate of processing (how quickly or slowly our brain processes information) (Knudsen 2007); and (4) assessing the degree of mental effort exerted (Bruya 2010). These functions are critical to self-regulation in everyday and skilled encounters (Powers 2010; Carver and Scheier 1981).

In cognitive science, attention is considered a limited resource (capacity) (Kahneman 1973). We 'pay' attention, implying that there is a mental price associated with attending (Sewall 1999: 18). We can only attend to so many things at once. Our capacity to attend is limited by the nature and amount (volume) of information, the capacity of working memory and many other features that may or not be relevant to the task at hand (Van Merriënboer and Sweller 2005; Paas, Renkel and Sweller 2004; Van Merriënboer and Sweller 2010). This speaks to the importance of designing instructional formats that support learner characteristics (Leppink et al. 2013). Tasks with a high degree of interactivity and multitasking, for example, tend toward higher cognitive loading – an important consideration for dance.

Finally, attention takes *mental* effort to keep information stable and focused (Csikszentmihalyi and Nakamura 2010: 182). The perception of effort is a complex phenomenon highly associated with attention control (Tang and Posner 2009; Ives and Shelley 2003; Ruehle and Zamansky 1997; Sarter, Gehring and Kozak 2006). Motivation, expectation, emotional threats or rewards and many other psychic phenomena compound the relationship between mental and physical effort (Kahneman 1973; Lamme and Roelfsema 2000; Sarter, Gehring and Kozak 2006; van Gaal et al. 2012). The degree to which one can *control* attention correlates with states of effortlessness and improved performance

(Csikszentmihalyi 1990). Mental effort tends to increase as demands to improve performance increase, or performing conditions remain unduly challenging.

Effortlessness in skilled performance is defined as a psychophysical state where 'movement flows automatically and flawlessly…relatively free of excessive mental or physical effort' (Dietrich and Stoll 2010:159, 160). Generally, the degree of 'attentional effort' is associated with task difficulty (Sarter, Gehring and Kozak 2006: 147). In building physical skills, learners aim to evolve from more effortful phases of learning to effortless mastery. Exercise physiologists measure effort in perceived exertion (Borg 1962), as well as in metabolic terms (Backs and Seljos 1994). Since the 1960s, the Borg scale has been the gold standard for measuring the subjective perception of effort in physical exercise (Borg 1962). Scientists can measure the degree of physical effort in terms of calories consumed. The subjective experience of physical or mental effort, however, is not automatically correlated with actual physiological output (see Batson 2013 for review). No one psychometric inventory differentiates mental from physical perception of effort (Rubio, Diaz, Martin and Puente 2004). Nor have neural pathways been mapped for effort in performing any task (Wulf and Lewthwaite 2010).

Attention and effort: the view from sports science

In sports science/psychology, attention training is designed to induce 'the performance enhancing state of mind' (Dietrich and Stoll 2010: 162). This 'state' is one where physical coordination approaches optimal levels of skilled control (Nielsen and Cohen 2008; Yarrow, Brown and Krakauer 2009; Wulf, McNevin and Shea 2001; Wulf 2007; Bruya 2010). Training aims at lowering the cost of performance while maximizing the benefits (a costs:benefits ratio) (Yarrow, Brown and Krakauer 2009). Dance scientists might frame the issue similarly: can attention training lower the psychophysical toll on the dancer while increasing the objective and subjective expectations for achievement? Performance expectations in dance might include efficiency and effectiveness in tangible or measurable qualities (such as accuracy of form, speed, balance etc.), as well as empathic expressiveness and communication of less tangible qualities (such as affective and aesthetic sensibility) (Krasnow and Chatfield 2009).

Performance adds many additional stresses to those encountered in everyday life. Dance scientists have described a number of factors that impact negatively on performance, such as anxiety, perfectionism and eating disorders (Nordin-Bates et al. 2011). Negative training environments (and/or personality traits) can hinder performance by rendering a dancer overly self-conscious, self-critical and preoccupied with making mistakes. Dancers exercise many self-regulatory strategies in coping with these kinds of stresses.[7] Like elite athletes, dance artists are known to handle the stresses of performance by delaying gratification, resisting distraction, inhibiting emotional outbreaks, giving themselves pep talks and sticking to task without recognizable rewards much longer than novice dancers. While not specific to attention training, these skills are interrelated. They impact positively on goal-setting, self-efficacy, self-confidence and other skills that impact on performance success (Nordin Bates et al. 2011).

A number of general skills of attentional control practiced in sports are also practiced in dance. Athletes and dancers often thrive in a team environment. Both attend not only to their own movements but also to those of other players/dancers at large. Skill depends on how quickly, easily and readily the player/dancer can select from the amount of stimuli coming from body, environment and task demands (cognitive load and rate of processing), while readily ignoring irrelevant stimuli. At the same time, constraints on a dancer's attention differ from those of an athlete. These constraints include the choreographer's aesthetic goals, the realistic necessities of performance in terms of time and resources, the dancer's personal factors and goals, the material constraints of practice/performance and other factors. Moment-by-moment challenges are dictated not by the need to win a game (although dance competitions might be subject to similar stresses), but by aesthetic concerns (Cross and Ticini 2012; Bläsing et al. 2012). Aesthetic demands take priority. The foregrounding of bodily expression requires kinesthetic nuance to project and enhance communication (Hawkins 1992; Debono 2004). Attending to one's own movements within the changing dynamics of the whole takes on another dimension. Attention is often linked to decision-making around contingencies that are emergent – instantaneously goal-less within a larger structure of movement creation. Here, for example, dancers may suspend personal goals to be part of the creative process (deLahunta, Barnard and McGregor 2009).

Training approaches

Attention is amenable to training. Training attention in the culture of western science is designed to expand capabilities as well as remediate problems (Figure 6.1). In sports- and cognitive psychology, for example, a number of methods strive to help persons achieve more optimal states of mind. These ideally also help improve physical (i.e., athletic) performance. The general aim is to induce a more focused and relaxed state of mind in order to attend without excess anxiety and distraction. Trainees exercise a number of different mental strategies to help keep focused while avoiding distracting elements. In athletics, attention training is geared first toward quickly identifying the locus of the problem(s) – personal characteristics, task demands or the environment context. Second, the training teaches the athlete to correct these problems either on the spot or in advance of their occurrence (Gill 2000).

In sports, much of the success of these trainings appears associated with the athlete's level of skill. Elite athletes generally organize themselves far more efficiently (they require less brain energy) (Ross et al. 2003). They are more economical and more efficient in motor planning as well as in motor unit recruitment (Hatfield et al. 2004; Haufler et al. 2000; Lay et al. 2002). Results from brain-imaging and behavioral studies show that elite athletes learn more quickly and efficiently than novices, and their performance is more consistent over a wider range of environmental conditions (Fitts and Posner 1973). Elite athletes make decisions more quickly and appropriately. They readily predict their own errors, modifying them within the moment. Further, they readily engage complex strategies to deal with uncertainty (Yarrow, Brown and Krakauer 2009). These strategies appear as readily in actual game conditions as they do in practice, where anxiety and other factors are heightened. Highly trained athletes also reveal differences in neural (brain) activation compared with novices (sport and task being equal). They exhibit a decrease in the overall volume of brain activation with a concomitant increase in activation in brain regions specific to task execution (Jancke et al. 2000; Münte et al. 2002, 2003; Ross et al. 2003; Schlaug 2001).[8] Further, peripheral neuromuscular activity also shows a reduction in muscle fiber recruitment in key muscle groups (Lay et al. 2002). These findings suggest a reduction in excessive variability in movement patterns (Araujo, Davids and Hristovski 2006; Milton et al. 2004; Pelz 2000).

Training elements in sports simulate exercise prescriptions to a certain extent. Physical variables such as the mode, load, intensity, frequency, duration and time for recovery are adjusted for mental tasks and embedded in the protocol. Cognitive psychology offers a broad range of behavioral therapies as well. Trainings can emphasize contemplative/meditative techniques as well as techniques for psychological coping and problem-solving. These self-regulatory strategies enhance focus by modulating thoughts, emotions and behaviors (Behncke 2002). Differences in trainings exist in philosophy as well as outcome. Western styles of attention training more readily exercise mental effort. While results may transfer to other cognitive abilities, this kind of training tends to produce mental fatigue (Tang and Posner 2009). Approaches deriving from eastern philosophical traditions tend toward attaining a state of effortlessness through training *mindfulness.* Western-style mental practice is designed to alter neural 'networks associated with cognitive tasks'. Eastern approaches, on the other hand, seek to 'achieve a state leading to more efficient self-regulation' (Tang and Posner 2009: 222).

Mindfulness training (Kabat-Zinn 1979: 1990) is usually taught in contemplative conditions (sitting quietly), requiring focusing awareness of body and mind on the present moment and directing or redirecting awareness toward staying present (Shapiro et al. 2008; Dijkstra, Kaschak and Zwaan 2007). Mindful approaches engage the autonomic nervous system in aiming to achieve a relaxed and balanced state, which transfers not only to cognition alone, but also to emotion and social behaviors (Tang and Posner 2009). These approaches more readily include physical practices, such as yoga and tai chi. At present, little is known about the comparative effectiveness of two approaches on the general population (Shapiro et al. 2008; Walsh and Shapiro 2006), nor of their effects on sports or dance.

What kind of attention training best enhances dance performance? Obviously, each and every dance context demands separate analysis (Caspersen 2011). Dance itself is the primary means for training skills of attention. Through dance praxis, dancers ideally learn to remove psychophysical interferences in order to allow dance to happen. To quote choreographer Deborah Hay: 'The dance lets me know what it is. I try to stay out of it as much as possible' (Hay 2004). A fine line exists, however, between the serendipitous emergence of mental/

physical effortlessness and cultivating these skills on one's own. How can dancers attend to the demands of technique and choreography without interfering with movement potential in the demanded skill? How much control is voluntary? What if the dancer's skills of embodied attention need re-education? What can a dancer do if interferences derail attention and become unmanageable? What if psychophysical interferences are simply overwhelming and the dancer cannot steer attention toward more optimal goals?

Somatic training

In dance, attention is trained extensively through an array of mindful and embodied movement practices. These occur in many contexts and milieus throughout the dancer's career – both within formal dance – and supplemental trainings, including Somatics. In Somatics (and somatically informed dance), attention training assumes a phenomenological dimension. Two basic somatic skills are attention and intention, out of which all other complex emotions and actions emerge (Gold 1992/93). More fundamentally, attention is essential to developing a flexible ongoing conversation between bodily states and gravity.[9] The moving, expressing body becomes the embodied 'interface' (Latour 2004: 205) between self and context. Here, body and context 'are tools of apprehension as well as of action' (Bar-On Cohen 2006 87). They are interwoven and reciprocal processes of self-regulation (Juhan 1986).

Self-regulatory skills rarely are achieved by imposing rigid methods of self-talk and control without paying a price (an increase in mental-physical fatigue and a decrease in coordination, for example). Among the possible models for training, some suggest a shift away from conditioning models toward more somatic movement-based techniques (Batson and Schwartz 2007) or more mindful ones (Lalitaraja 2012). Visualization, imagination, empathic communication and, of course, movement, are integral to the quality of attention. All these 'facilitate apprehension and navigation of the bodyscape' (Hawksley 2011: 108) in learning environments that encourage an exploratory, experiential, reflective atmosphere. Here, any one sensory (or other systems) or behavioral mode of engagement may focus the attention on key variables within the moving gestalt.

In martial arts, repeated practice is considered key to learning to attune to the subtleties of effort underlying bodymind coordination. As karate student Bar-On Cohen describes: The 'way' of training is through 'repeating movements over and over again until perfect praxis can be approached, while progressing smoothly, without high points, interruptions or intervals within the body' (Bar-On Cohen 2006: 77). It is important to emphasize, however, that it is not mere repetition alone that makes the difference. Rather, it is through attending to the *subtleties* of embodied sensation within repeated practice that bodies are 'constructed anew' (ibid.: 74).

The meaning of the teacher's words, the ways in which an exercise is carried out, and ultimately karate itself, emerge from within an individual's body. But how can the body, perceived and "operated" as it is from within, be culturally transmitted? How can internal somatic experiences originate from without?…The long process of discovering karate inside one's body also involves words…Those words are meaningless to a beginner, but they become gradually loaded with significance, and their meaning shifts as the student's understanding of them is modified through somatic experience. I call such words, whose deciphering depends on somatic experience and whose meaning varies accordingly, "somatic codes". Somatic codes verbalize interior body dynamics, and their significance emerges together with these dynamics…Somatic codes are neither "out there" nor "in here"; they are both in the world and part of me, of my body…[their] emergence depends on interaction, and it is also a tool of interaction, a social instrument that can be put to use inter-subjectively.

(ibid.: 74–75)

Likewise in dance, attention is linked intimately to the practice of attending to the dynamics of the moving bodymind (Clarke, Kramer and Müller 2010). Understanding the interrelationship between attention and effortlessness necessitates developing 'empirical methods as process' (Clarke, Kramer and Müller 2010: 205). These may differ from sports, martial arts or other psychophysical practices. Dance is an explication of empathic, communicative art (Warburton 2011). The kind of poly-attentional flexibility differs from other physical practices. Attentional focus is harnessed at any one time to multiple demands of body expressivity within the dance context. Each action – each phase of dance praxis – shifts the nature and degree of focus (Bläsing et al. 2012).

Contemporary dance teacher and British dancemaker Gill Clarke has written about the multiple somatic approaches to training attention in her dance classes (deLahunta, Clarke and Barnard 2012).[10] Clarke suggests that the '[f]lexibility, variability, and effort expressivity towards choreographic goals' [requires] 'tuning the mind, the body, and the imagination as one thing…' (Clarke, Kramer and Müller 2010: 203). The dancer attends to the changing valences of internal and external cues. These cues arise against the continually changing background of demands and goals within the dance, and the momentary salience of expressive body.

Dancemaker Sue Hawksley notes that dancers 'may be called upon to be singularly or simultaneously aware of their in-depth body, of peripersonal space, of inter-personal space between self-co-performers and the performance environment, of projection to an audience, of extension through virtual environments, and distantiation from oneself through adopting a character or generating an external viewpoint as if from the audience's perspective' (Hawsley 2011: 102). Hawksley suggests that training 'attentional alacrity' is key in facilitating 'an attitude of embodied reflection and skills of perceptual awareness' that lead to 'performance *as* practice and practices *for* performance' (ibid.: 102). The performative environment, too, is a physical, emotional and aesthetic gestalt in constant flux. Attention and decision-making are tethered to what dancing is and demands, even when the goals are improvisational (Kampe 2010). Attention is shaped by the variability, vividness, degree of absorption within the context and, perhaps, even the inclusion of reflective experience within the experience.

In conclusion, somatically informed dance offers many other examples of how body, mind and context work together toward unleashing movement potential, freedom and mastery. Greater insight into the performative bodymind is possible, as researchers continue to examine attention and effort in dance praxis. More questions than answers arise at this point. The next three chapters re-examine somatic education as exemplifying embodied cognitive approaches to understanding this mysterious relationship.

Explorations for this chapter appear in Appendix II.

References

Anderson, John R. (2004), *Cognitive Psychology and its Implications,* 6 edn, New York, NY: Worth Publishers.

Araujo, D., Davids, K. and Hristovski, R. (2006), 'The ecological dynamics of decision making in sport', *Psychology of Sport and* Exercise, 7: 6, pp. 653–76.

Arvidson, P.S. (2003), 'A lexicon of attention: From cognitive science to phenomenology', *Phenomenology and the Cognitive Sciences*, 2: 2, 99–132.

Arvidson, P.S. (2010), 'Attention in context' in D. Schmicking and S. Gallagher (eds.), *Handbook of Phenomenology and Cognitive Science*, New York, NY: Springer, pp. 99–121.

Ashbury, C. and Rich, B. (2008), 'Learning, arts, and the brain: The Dana Consortium report on arts and cognition', New York, NY: Dana Foundation.

Backs, R.W. and Seljos, K.A. (1994), 'Metabolic and cardiorespiratory measures of mental effort: The effects of level of difficulty in a working memory task', *International Journal of Psychophysiology*, 16: 1, pp. 57–68.

Balgaonkar, A.V. (2010), 'Effect of dance/motor therapy on the cognitive development of children', *International Journal of Arts and Sciences*, 3: 11, pp. 54–72.

Bargh, J.A. and Chartrand, T.L. (1999), 'The unbearable automaticity of being', *American Psychologist*, 54: 7, pp. 462–79.

Bar-On Cohen, E. (2006), 'Kime and the moving body: Somatic codes in Japanese martial arts', *Body and Society*, 12: 4, pp. 73–93.

Bari, A. and Robbins, T.W. (2013), 'Inhibition and impulsivity: Behavioral and neural basis of response control', *Progress in Neurobiology*, 108, pp. 44–79.

Batson, G. and Schwartz, R.E. (2007), 'Revisiting the value of somatic education in dance training through an inquiry into practice schedules', *Journal of Dance Education*, 7: 2, pp. 47–57.

Batson, G. (2009), 'The somatic practice of intentional rest in dance education – preliminary steps towards a method of study', *Journal of Dance and Somatic Practices*, 1: 2, pp. 177–97.

Batson, G. (2013), 'Exercise-induced central fatigue: A review of the literature with implications for dance science research', *Journal of Dance Medicine and Science*, 17: 2, pp. 53–62.

Bauer, P.J. and Zelazo, P.D. (2013), 'The NIH toolbox cognition battery: Summary, conclusions, and implications for cognitive development', *Monographs of the Society for Research in Child Development*, 78: 4, pp. 133–46.

Blaser, P. and Hökelman, A. (2009), 'Mental reproduction of a dance choreography and its effects on physiological fatigue in dancers', *Journal of Human Sport and Exercise,*

4: 2, pp. 129–41. http://www.jhse.ua.es/jhse/article/view/54/144. Accessed 18 September 2013.

Bläsing, B., Calvo-Merino, B., Cross, E.S., Jola, C., Honisch, J. and Stevens, C.J. (2012), 'Neurocognitive control in dance perception and performance', *Acta Psychologica*, 139, pp. 300–08.

Behncke, L. (2002), 'Self-regulation', *Athletic Insight: The Online Journal of Sports Psychology*. http://www.athleticinsight.com/Vol4Iss1/SelfRegulation.htm. Accessed 12 September 2012.

Borg, G. (1962), *Physical Performance and Perceived Exertion*, Lund: C.W.K. Gleerup.

Bruya, B. (ed.) (2010), *Effortless Attention: A New Perspective in the Cognitive Science of Attention and Action*, Cambridge, MA: MIT Press.

Buchanan, P.A. and Ulrich, B.D. (2001), 'The Feldenkrais Method: A dynamic approach to changing motor behavior', *Research Quarterly for Exercise and Sport*, 72: 4, pp. 315–23.

Cabeza, R. and Nyberg, L. (1997), 'Imaging cognition: An empirical review of PET studies with normal subjects', *Journal of Cognitive Neuroscience*, 9: 1, pp. 1–26.

Carver, C.S. and Scheier, M.F. (1981), 'The self-attention-induced feedback loop and social facilitation', *Journal of Experimental Social Psychology*, 17: 6, pp. 545–68.

Caspersen, D. (2011), 'Decreation: Fragmentation and unity' in S. Spier (ed.), *William Forsythe and the Practice of Choreography: It Starts From Any Point*, London: Routledge, pp. 93–100.

Chan, R.C.K., Shum, D., Toulopoulou, T. and Chen, E. (2008), 'Assessment of executive functions: Review of instruments and identification of critical issues', *Archives of Clinical Neuropsychology*, 23: 2, pp. 201–16.

Clarke, G., Cramer, F. and Müller, G. (2010), 'Minding motion' in I. Diehl and F. Lampert (eds.), *Dance Techniques 2010*, Leipzig: Henschel Verlag, pp. 199–229.

Coubard, O.A., Duretz, S., Lefebvre, V., Lapalus, P. and Ferrunfino, L. (2011), 'Practice of contemporary dance improves cognitive flexibility', *Frontiers in Aging Neuroscience*, 3: 3, pp. 1–14.

Coubard, O. A., Duretz, S., Lefebvre, V., Lapalus, P. and Ferrufino, L. (2011), 'Practice of contemporary dance improves cognitive flexibility in aging', *Frontiers in Aging Neuroscience*, 3. http://www.frontiersin.org/Journal/10.3389/fnagi.2011.00013/abstract. Accessed 15 October 2013.

Cross, E.S. and Ticini, L.F. (2012), 'Neuroaesthetics and beyond: New horizons in applying the science of the brain to the art of dance', *Phenomenology and the Cognitive Sciences*, 11: 1, pp. 5–16.

Csikszentmihalyi, M. (1975), *Beyond Boredom and Anxiety: Experiencing Flow in Work and Play*, San Francisco, CA: Jossey-Bass.

Cszikszentmihalyi, M. (1990), *Flow: The Psychology of Optimal Experience*, New York, NY: HarperCollins.

Csikszentmihalyi, M. (1993), *The Evolving Self: A Psychology for the Third Millennium*, New York, NY: Harper Perennial.

Cszikszentmihalyi, M. and Nakamura, J. (2010), 'Effortless attention in everyday life' in B. Bruya (ed.), *Effortless Attention: A New Perspective in the Cognitive Science of Attention and Action*, Cambridge, MA: MIT Press, pp. 179–89.

Debono, M.-W. (2004), 'From perception to consciousness: An epistemic vision of evolutionary processes', *Leonardo*, 37: 3, pp. 243–48.

Dehaene, S. and Naccache, L. (2001), 'Towards a cognitive neuroscience of consciousness: Basic evidence and a workspace framework', *Cognition*, 79, pp. 1–37.

deLahunta, S., Barnard, P. and McGregor, W. (2009), 'Augmenting choreography: Using insights and inspiration from science' in J. Butterworth and L. Wildschut (eds.), *Contemporary Choreography: A Critical Reader*, New York, NY: Routledge, pp. 431–48.

deLahunta, S., Clarke, G. and Barnard, P. (2012), 'A conversation about choreographic thinking tools', *Journal of Dance and Somatic Practices*, 3: 1–2, pp. 243–59.

Dietrich, A. and Stoll, O. (2010), 'Effortless attention, hypofrontality, and perfectionism' in B. Bruya (ed.), *Effortless Attention: A New Perspective in the Cognitive Science of Attention and Action*, Cambridge, MA: MIT Press, pp. 159–78.

Dijkstra, K., Kaschak, M.P. and Zwaan, A. (2007), 'Body posture facilitates retrieval of autobiographical memories', *Cognition*, 102, pp. 139–49.

Dormashev, Y. (2010), 'Flow experience explained on the grounds of an activity approach to attention' in B. Bruya (ed.), *Effortless Attention: A New Perspective in the Cognitive Science of Attention and Action*, Cambridge, MA: MIT Press, pp. 287–334.

Fehmi, L. and Robbins, J. (2007), *The Open-Focus Brain: Harnessing the Power of Attention to Heal Mind and Body*, Boston, MA: Trumpeter Press.

Feldenkrais, M. (1964), 'Mind and body' in E. Beringer (ed.), *Embodied Wisdom, the Collected Papers of Moshe Feldenkrais*, Berkeley, CA: North Atlantic Books, p. 43.

Ferrufino, F., Bril, B., Dietrich, G., Nonaka, T. and Coubard, O.A. (2008), 'Practice of contemporary dance promotes stochastic postural control in aging', *Frontiers in Human Neuroscience*, http://www.frontiersin.org/human_neuroscience/10.3389/fnhum.2011.00169/ abstract. Accessed 14 February 2013.

Fitts, P and Posner, M. (1973), *Human Performance*, London: Prentice-Hall.

Giguere, M. (2011), 'Social influences on the creative process: An examination of children's creativity and learning in dance', *International Journal of Education and the Arts*, 12: 1.5. http://www.ijea.org/v12si1/v12si1-5.pdf. Accessed 18 January 2013.

Gill, D.L. (2000), *Psychological Dynamics of Sport and Exercise* (2nd edn),Champaign, IL: Human Kinetics.

Gold, L. (1992/1993), 'Gaining grace – a somatic perspective', *Somatics*, 9: 1, pp. 34–39, online http://www.somatics.com/gold.htm#publications. Accessed 11 February 2011.

Green Gilbert, A. (2006), *Brain-Compatible Dance Education*, Arlington, VA: American Alliance for Health, Physical Education, Recreation and Dance.

Grove, R., Stevens, C. and McKechnie, S. (2005), *Thinking in Four Dimensions: Creativity and Cognition in Contemporary Dance*, Melbourne, AU: University of Melbourne Press.

Gruszka, A., Matthews, G. and Szymura, B. (eds.) (2010), *Handbook of Individual Differences in Cognition: Attention, Memory, and Executive Control*, New York, NY: Springer.

Gurwitsch, A. (1964), *The Field of Consciousness*, Pittsburgh, PA: Duquesne University Press.

Hanlon Johnson, D. (2000), 'Intricate tactile sensitivity: A key variable in Western integrative bodywork', *Progress in Brain Research*, 122, 479–90.

Hanlon Johnson, D. (2004), 'Body practices and human inquiry: Disciplined experiencing, fresh thinking and vigorous language' in J. Murphy, L. Esposito and V. Berdayes (eds.), *The Body in Human Inquiry: Interdisciplinary Explorations of Embodiment*, New York, NY: The Hampton Press.

Hanna, J.L. (2008), 'A nonverbal language for imagining and learning: Dance education in K–12 curriculum', *Educational Researcher*, 37: 8, pp. 491–506.

Hanna, T. (1990/91), 'Clinical somatic education: A new discipline in the field of health care', *Somatics, Magazine-Journal of the Bodily Arts and Sciences*, 8: 1. http://www.somatics.com/hannart.htm. Accessed 26 August 2013.

Harper, D. (2001–03), *Online Etymological Dictionary*, http://www.etymonline.com/index.php?term=attend. Accessed 30 September 2013.

Hatfield, B.D., Haufler, A.J., Hung, T.-M. and Spalding, T.W. (2004), 'Electroencephalographic studies of skilled psychomotor performance', *Journal of Clinical Neurophysiology*, 21: 3, pp. 144–56.

Haufler, A.J., Spalding, T.W., Santa Maria, D.L. and Hatfield, B.D. (2000), 'Neuro-cognitive activity during a self-paced visuospatial task: Comparative EEG profiles in marksmen and novice shooters', *Biological Psychology*, 53: 2–3, pp. 131–60.

Hawkins, E. (1992), *The Body Is a Clear Place: And Other Statements on Dance*, Princeton, NJ: Princeton Book Company.

Hawksley, S. (2011), 'Choreographic and somatic strategies for navigating bodyscapes and tensegrity schemata', *Journal of Dance and Somatic Practices*, 3: 1–2, pp. 101–10.

Hay, D. (2004), 'A Lecture on the performance of beauty', http://www.deborahhay.com/scores_lecture_beauty.html. Accessed 14 February 2013.

Hossner, E.-J. and Wenderoth, N. (eds.) (2009), 'Gabriele Wulf on attentional focus and motor learning', *E Journal Bewegung und Training*, 1, pp. 1–74. http://www.sportwissenschaft.de/fileadmin/pdf/BuT/hossner_wulf.pdf. Accessed 14 February 2013.

Ives, J.C. and Shelley, G.A. (2003), 'Psychophysics in functional strength and power training: Review and implementation framework', *Journal of Strength and Conditioning Research*, 17: 1, pp. 177–86.

Jackson, S.A., Thomas, P.R., Marsh, H.W. and Smethurst, C.J. (2001), 'Relationships between flow, self-concept, psychological skills and performance', *Journal of Applied Sport Psychology*, 13, pp. 129–153.

James, W. (1890), *The Principles of Psychology*, Vol. 1, New York, NY: Henry Holt, pp. 403–44.

Jancke, L., Shahb, N.J. and Peters, M. (2000), 'Cortical activations in primary and secondary motor areas for complex bimanual movements in professional pianists', *Cognitive Brain Research*, 10, pp. 177–83.

Jovancevic, J., Rosano, C., Perera, S., Erickson, K. and Studenski, S. (2012), 'A protocol for a randomized clinical trial of interactive video dance: Potential for effects on cognitive function', *BioMedCentral Geriatrics*. http://www.biomedcentral.com/1471-2318/12/23. Accessed 20 December 2012.

Juhan, D. (1987), *Job's Body: A Handbook for Bodyworkers*, Barrytown, NY: Stationhill Press.

Kabat-Zinn, J. (1979), 'The Stress Reduction Program', http://www.umassmed.edu/cfm/stress/index.aspx. Accessed 25 August 2013.

Kabat-Zinn, J. (1990), *Full Catastrophe Living: Using the Wisdom of Your Mind to Face Stress, Pain and Illness*, New York, NY: Dell Publishing.

Kahneman, D. (1973), *Attention and Effort*, Englewood Cliffs, NJ: Prentice-Hall.

Kampe, T. (2010), '"Weave": The Feldenkrais Method as Choreographic Process', *Performio*, 1: 2, pp. 34–52.

Kattenstroth, J.-C., Kolankowska, I., Kalisch, T. and Dinse, H.R. (2010), 'Superior sensory, motor, and cognitive performance in elderly individuals with multi-year dancing activities', *Frontiers in Aging Neuroscience*, 2: 31, pp. 1–9.

Kattenstroth, J.-C., Kalisch, T., Kolankowska, I. and Dinse, H.R. (2011), 'Balance, sensorimotor, and cognitive performance in long-year expert senior ballroom dancers', *Journal of Aging Research*, http://www.hindawi.com/journals/jar/2011/176709/. Accessed 22 September 2013.

Kattenstroth, J.-C., Kalisch, T., Holt, S., Tegenthoff, M. and Dinse, H.R. (2013), 'Six months of dance intervention enhances postural, sensorimotor, and cognitive performance in elderly without affecting cardio-respiratory functions', *Frontiers in Aging Neuroscience*, 4, pp. 35–44.

Keinänen, M., Hetland, L. and Winner, E. (2000), 'Teaching cognitive skill through dance: Evidence for near but not far transfer', *Journal of Aesthetic Education*, 34: 3/4, pp. 295–306.

Kim, S.-H., Kim, M., Yu-Bae, A., Lim, H.-K. et al. (2011), 'Effect of dance exercise on cognitive function in elderly patients with metabolic syndrome: A pilot study', *Journal of Sports Science and Medicine*, 10, pp. 617–78.

Kinchia, R.A. (1980), 'The measurement of attention' in R.S. Nickerson (ed.), *Attention and Performance VIII*, International Association for the Study of Attention and Performance, Hillsdale, NJ: Lawrence Erlbaum Associates.

Knudsen, E.I. (2007), 'Fundamental components of attention', *Annual Review of Neuroscience*, 30: 1, pp. 57–78.

Krasnow, D. and Chatfield, S.J. (2009), 'Development of the "Performance Competence Evaluation Measure": Assessing qualitative aspects of dance performance', *Journal of Dance Medicine and Science*, 13: 4, pp. 101–07.

Lalitaraja, J.C. (2012), 'A Buddhist's approach to choreography as spiritual practice', *Journal of Dance and Somatic Practices*, 4: 1, pp. 143–54.

Lamme, V.A. and Roelfsema, P.R. (2000), 'The distinct modes of vision offered by feedforward and recurrent processing', *Trends in Cognitive Neurosciences*, 23: 11, pp. 571–79.

Latour, B. (2004), 'How to talk about the body', *Body & Society*, 10: 2–3, pp. 205–29.

Lay, B.S., Sparrow, W.A., Hughes, K.M. and O'Dwyer, N.J. (2002), 'Practice effects on coordination and control, metabolic energy expenditure, and muscle activation', *Human Movement Science*, 21: 5–6, pp. 807–30.

Leppink, J., Paas, F., Van der Vleuten, C.P., Van Gog, T. and Van Merrienboer, J.J. (2013), 'Development of an instrument for measuring different types of cognitive load', *Behavioral Research* (ahead of print).

Leri, D. (1997). 'Mental furniture#10. The Fechner Weber Law', *Semiophysics*, http://www.semiophysics.com/SemioPhysics_Articles_mental_10.html. Accessed 25 August 2013.

Mangun, G.R. (2011), *Neuroscience of Attention: Attentional Control and Selection.* Cambridge, MA: Oxford University Press.

Milton, J., Small, S. and Solodkin, A. (2004), 'On the road to automatic: Dynamic aspects of skill acquisition', *Journal of Clinical Neurophysiology*, 21: 3, pp. 134–43.

Milton, J., Solodkin, A., Hlustik, P. and Small, S.J. (2007), 'The mind of expert motor performance is cool and focused', *NeuroImage*, 35, pp. 804–13.

Moffett, A.-T. (2012), 'Higher order thinking in the dance studio', *Journal of Dance Education*, 12, pp. 1–6.

Mole, C. (2013). 'Attention', *Stanford Encyclopedia of Philosophy*, http://plato.stanford.edu/entries/attention/. Accessed 25 August 2013.

Moller, A.C., Meier, B.P. and Wall, R.D. (2010), 'Developing an experimental induction of flow: Effortless action in the lab' in B. Bruya (ed.), *Effortless Attention: A New Perspective in the Cognitive Science of Attention and Action*, Cambridge, MA: MIT Press, pp. 159–78.

Moore, M., Drake, D., Tschannen-Moran, B., Campone, F. and Kauffman, C. (2005), 'Relational Flow: A Theoretical Model for the Intuitive Dance', Coaching Research Symposium, San Jose, CA. http://free-doc-lib.com/book/relational-flow-a-theoretical-model-for-the-intuitive-dance.pdf. Accessed 10 January 2013.

Münte, T.F., Altermuller, E. and Janckle, L. (2002), 'The musician's brain as a model of neuroplasticity', *Nature Reviews Neuroscience*, 3: 6, pp. 473–78.

Münte, T.F., Nager, W., Beiss, T., Schroeder, C. and Altenmüller, E. (2003), 'Specialization of the specialized: Electrophysiological investigations in professional musicians', *Annals of the New York Academy of Sciences*, 999, pp. 131–39.

Muraven, M., Tice, D.M. and Baumeister, R.F. (1998), 'Self-control as limited resource: Regulatory depletion patterns', *Personality and Social Psychology,* 74: 3, pp. 774–89.

Nakamura, J. and Csikszentmihalyi, M. (2002), 'The concept of flow' in C. R. Snyder and S.J. Lopez (eds.), *Handbook of Positive Psychology*, New York, NY: Oxford University Press, pp. 89–105.

Nielsen, J.B. and Cohen, J. (2008), 'The Olympic brain: Does corticospinal plasticity play a role in the acquisition of skills required for high-performance sports?', *Journal of Physiology*, 586: 1, pp. 65–70.

Nordin-Bates, S., Cumming, J., Aways, D. and Sharp, L. (2011), 'Imagining yourself dancing to perfection? Correlates of perfectionism among ballet and contemporary dancers', *Journal of Clinical Sport Psychology*, 5, pp. 58–76.

Paas, F., Renkel, A. and Sweller, J. (2004), 'Cognitive load theory: Instructional implications of the interaction between information structures and cognitive architecture', *Instructional Science*, 32, pp. 1–8.

Peh, S.Y.C., Chow, J.Y. and Davids, K. (2011), 'Focus of attention and its impact on movement behaviour', *Journal of Science and Medicine in Sport*, 14: 1, pp. 70–78.

Pelz, D. (2000), *Dave Pelz's Putting Bible*, New York, NY: Doubleday.

Pickens, S., Ostwald S.K., Murphy-Pace, K. and Bergstrom N. (2010), 'Systematic review of current executive function measures in adults with and without cognitive impairments', *International Evidence Based Healthcare*, 8: 3: pp. 110–25.

Powers, R. (2010). 'Use it or lose it: Dancing makes you smarter', http://socialdance.stanford.edu/syllabi/smarter.htm. Accessed 24 August 2013.

Posner, M.I. and Rothbart, M.K. (1998), 'Attention, self-regulation and consciousness', *Philosophical Transactions of the Royal Society of London B*, 353, pp. 1915–27.

Posner, M.I. and Patoine, B. (2009). 'How arts training improves attention and cognition', *Dana News*, The Dana Foundation. http://dana.org/news/cerebrum/detail.aspx?id=23206. Accessed 10 December 2012.

Rubio, S., Díaz, E., Martín, J. and Puente, J.M. (2004), 'Evaluation of subjective mental workload: A comparison of SWAT, NASA-TLX, and workload profile methods', *Applied Psychology*, 53: 1, pp. 61–86.

Ruehle, B.L. and Zamansky, H.S. (1997), 'The experience of effortlessness in hypnosis: Perceived or real?', *International Journal of Clinical and Experimental Hypnosis*, 45: 2, pp. 144–57.

Ross, J.S., Thach, J., Ruggieri, P.M., Lieber, M. and Lapresto, E. (2003), 'The mind's eye: Functional MR imaging evaluation of golf motor imagery', *American Journal of Neurological Radiology*, 24: 6, pp. 1036–44.

Sarter, M., Gehring, W.J. and Kozak, R. (2006), 'More attention must be paid: The neurobiology of attentional effort', *Brain Research Reviews*, 51, pp. 45–160.

Schlaug, G. (2006), 'The brain of musicians: A model for functional and structural adaptation', *Annals of the New York Academy of Sciences*, 930, pp. 281–99.

Schmeichel, B.J. and Baumeiser, R.F. (2010), 'Effortful attention control' in B. Bruya (ed.), *Effortless Attention: A New Perspective in the Cognitive Science of Attention and Action*, Cambridge, MA: MIT Press, pp. 29–51.

Schmidt, L. (2011), 'Toward an enactive approach to hearing media', *The Sound Track*, 4: 1, pp. 33–42.

Sewell, L. (1999), *Sight and Sensibility: The Ecological Psychology of Seeing*, New York, NY: Jeremy P. Tarcher.

Shapiro, S.L., Oman, D., Thoresen, C.E., Plante, T.G. and Flinders, T. (2008), 'Cultivating mindfulness: effects on well-being', *Journal of Clinical Psychology*, 64, pp. 840–62.

Sheets-Johnstone, M. (2010), 'Body and movement: Basic dynamic principles' in S. Gallagher and D. Schmicking (eds.), *Handbook of Phenomenology and Cognitive Science*, New York, NY: Springer, pp. 217–34.

Sheets-Johnstone, M. (2011), *The Primacy of Movement*, expanded 2nd edn, Philadelphia, PA: John Benjamin's Publishing Company.

Simonton, D.K. (2007), 'Creativity: Specialized expertise or general cognitive processes?' in M. J. Roberts (ed.), *Integrating the Mind: Domain General vs. Domain Specific Processes in Higher Cognition*, New York, NY: Psychology Press, pp. 351–68.

Stevens, C. and McKechnie, S. (2005), 'Minds and motion: Dynamical systems in choreography, creativity, and dance' in J. Birringer and J. Fenger (eds.), *Tanz im Kopf: Yearbook 15 of the German Dance Research Society*, Münster: LIT Verlag, pp. 241–52.

Tang, Y.-Y. and Posner, M.E. (2009), 'Attention training and attention state training', *Trends in Cognitive Sciences*, 13: 5, pp. 222–27.

Taylor, J. (2011), 'Dance articles: The Performing Attitude', http://drjimtaylor.com/2.0/dance/. Accessed 24 August 2013.

Thompson, E. (2010), *Mind in Life: Biology, Phenomenology and the Sciences of Mind*, Cambridge, MA: Harvard University Press.

Thompson, E. and Stapleton, M. (2008), 'Making sense of sense-making: Reflections on enactive and extended mind theories', *Topoi*, 28: 1, pp. 23–30.

Tye, M. (2013), 'Qualia', *The Stanford Encyclopedia of Philosophy*, http://plato.stanford.edu/entries/qualia/. Accessed 21 September 2013.

van Gaal, S., de Lange, F.P. and Cohen, M.X. (2012), 'The role of consciousness in cognitive control and decision making', *Frontiers in Human Neuroscience*, 6: 121, pp. 1–14.

van Merriënboer, J.J.G. and Sweller, J. (2005), 'Cognitive load theory and complex learning: Recent developments and future directions', *Educational Psychology Review*, 17, pp. 147–77.

van Merrienboer, J.J.G. and Sweller, J. (2010), 'Cognitive load theory in health professional education: Design principles and strategies', *Medical Education*, 44, pp. 85–93.

Varela, F., Thompson, E. and Rosch, E. (1991), *The Embodied Mind: Cognitive Science and Human Experience*, Cambridge, MA: MIT Press.

Walsh, R. and Shapiro, S.L. (2006), 'The meeting of meditative disciplines and Western psychology: A mutually enriching dialogue', *American Psychologist*, 61, pp. 227–39.

Warburton, T.E. (2011), 'Of meanings and movements: Re-languaging embodiment in dance phenomenology and cognition', *Dance Research Journal*, 43: 2, pp. 65–83.

Wulf, G. (2007), *Attention and Motor Skill Learning*, Champaign, IL: Human Kinetics.

Wulf, G., McNevin, N. and Shea, C.H. (2001), 'The automaticity of complex motor skill learning as a function of attentional focus', *The Quarterly Journal of Experimental Psychology: Section A*, 54: 4, pp. 1143–54.

Wulf, G. and Lewthwaite, R. (2010), 'Effortless motor learning? An external focus of attention enhances movement effectiveness and efficiency' in B. Bruya (ed.), *Effortless Attention: A New Perspective in Attention and Action*, Cambridge, MA: MIT Press, pp. 75–101.

Yarrow, K., Brown, P. and Krakauer, J.W. (2009), 'Inside the brain of an elite athlete: The neural processes that support high achievement in sports', *Nature Reviews Neuroscience*, 10: 8, pp. 585–96.

Notes

1   In phenomenology, sensory qualities are referred to as qualia. For further reference, consult Tye (2013) and Sheets-Johnstone (2010; 2011).

2   Attention training is geared to improve mental and physical skills as well as to address deficits (such as attention deficit hyperactivity disorder). Emphasis in these trainings often relies on the concept of attention *control*, which has to do with aspects of focus, flexibility and handling anxiety. These approaches not only are comprised of video games and other computer-based programs, but also involve trips to nature camps or exposure to other natural environments. A number of neuroscience websites have cropped up in the last few years that offer a variety of cognitive approaches to improve attention control. For example, see http://www.teach-the-brain.org/; www.lumosity.com; www. sharpbrains.org; and http://www.positscience.com/.

3   Dance training is reputed to enhance cognitive faculties in children (Green Gilbert 2006; Hanna 2008) and adults (Keinänen, Hetland and Winner 2000), as well as improve academic achievement in a variety of subjects from English to statistics. See, for example, http://flraen.org/resources/article-archive/46-news/front-page/138-students-dance-to-improve-

their-english and http://www.openculture.com/2013/10/statistics-explained-with-modern-dance.html.

4   Of all the models linking attention and performance, perhaps the best known is Csikszentmihalyi's model of *flow*. Between the 1970s and 1990s, social psychologist Mihaly Csikszentmihalyi honed his theory of the phenomenology of 'flow', a subjective experience of effortlessness emerging when a person is fully engaged in an activity (Csikszentmihalyi 1975; 1990; Csikszentmihalyi and Nakamura 2010). Flow is an autotelic experience, a zone where persons are challenged at a high level of skill awareness to become *in synch* with an activity (Moore et al. 2005). Basically, the experience of flow is enjoyable and pleasurable, relatively free of anxiety, in which the performer feels a sense of efficacy, confidence and motivation to perform (Jackson et al. 2001). The state is described as a merging of action and awareness in which a deepening sense of engagement with the activity is balanced with ease of concentration, loss of reflective self-consciousness and an elevated sense of control and self-efficacy (Bruya 210: 186). The state engenders a comparatively different experience of self, a feeling of being in control with a concomitant sensation of physical and mental effortlessness, free of self-consciousness, and an altered sense of time (Bruya 2010: 5). In this state, people can act more autonomously and independently, because they are free of external threats of manipulation or dependent on external rewards (Csikszentmihalyi 1990). Csikszentmihalyi initially portrayed flow as a state in which one's perceived abilities were balanced by the perceived challenge at a high enough level to avoid both boredom (too much skill for the challenge) and anxiety (too much challenge for the skill). Ideally, a sense of effortlessness correlates not only with improved coordination and performance of the activity, but also with a feeling of enhanced benefits from doing the activity (Csikszentmihalyi 1990). Of interest, is the notion of *perceived* ability. Perceived skill level is not necessarily commensurate with actual skill level. '[I]t is not the skills we actually have that determine how we feel, but the ones we think we have' (Csikszentmihalyi 1990: 75). Clarity of goals and timely feedback play an enormous role (Moller, Meier and Wall 2010). Someone can more readily approach a state of flow when goals of the activity are clear (either implicitly or explicitly) and feedback is immediate (Csikszentmihalyi 1993; Nakamura and Csikszentmihalyi 2002).

5   Somatics offers many experiences in effortlessness and non-doing. Examples of consciously aware, movement trainings that underscore states of effortlessness include Ideokinesis, the Feldenkrais Method® and the Alexander Technique. Martial arts also aim at states of effortlessness, although practice environments differ, as they do in dance. Take the Feldenkrais Method® as an example of this kind of somatic learning approach. Moshe Feldenkrais' opening quote suggests that sensations of effort and coordination are intimately related – but *inversely*. The less the conscious perception of effort in movement, the more likely the mover is approaching a more coordinated state of bodymind unity. In formulating his somatic learning model back in the 1960s, Feldenkrais viewed attention not as a behavioral trait, but as a self-regulatory dynamic – flexible and adaptive through perceptual learning (Buchanan and Ulrich 2001). Moshe Feldenkrais modeled his Method˚ partly on the Fechner-Weber law of psychophysics (Leri 1997). Self-regulatory skills are trained through attending to sensory awareness of movement feedback. In many Awareness

Through Movement* lessons, for example, the learner attends to sensory feedback coming from verbally guided lessons for a prolonged period of time. The learner attempts to perform verbally directed movements as effortlessly as possible, attending to sensations (of effort and other sensory phenomena), as opposed to achieving movement goals. By attending to sensing and executing movements relatively free of goals, participants learn to move 'below the level of muscular achievement' normally associated with goal achievement (Hanna 1990/91). The result ideally is a reduction in unnecessary mental-physical effort in learning to move, resulting in the development of skill.

6   Authors Fehmi and Robbins (2007) suggest that a narrow focus of attention is largely rewarded in western culture. They offer a mental imagery-based program to correct this emphasis. See also sports science texts, such as Gill (2000) for chapters on attentional styles and training. Dancemakers can look to the work of Rudolph Laban and his descendants, certainly, for insights into attentional styles.

7   The term 'strategies' admittedly is mechanistic and does not convey the phenomenological depth of bodymind processing. This is also true of terms such as 'utility' and 'optimization'. These terms are, however, common within human movement science research.

8   In the pre-shot phase of golf, for example, the posterior cingulate, the amygdala–forebrain complex and the basal ganglia were active only in novices, whereas experts had activation primarily in the superior parietal lobule, the dorsal lateral premotor area and the occipital area. While this phase of golf allows the golfer the time to think, it is still interesting to see the higher activation of lower-level brain processes in the novices, compared with the elite golfers (Milton et al. 2007: 804). Novice golfers (presumably in a more immature stage of motor learning), show greater activation in the basal ganglia and the limbic system, which are areas normally activated in the brains of experts (Milton et al. 2007).

9   Many somatic practices train attention in unique ways. This idea of honing skills of attention as intrinsic to viable, lifelong development in gravity is elaborated in the work of Hubert Godard. See, for example, Newton (1995), 'Explorations: Basic concepts in the theory of Hubert Godard', http://www.resourcesinmovement.com/images/Articles/basic-conceptsHG.pdf.

10 Gill Clarke (1954–2011). Her obituary is located at http://www.theguardian.com/stage/2011/dec/20/gill-clarke.

Chapter 7

Training Attention - The Somatic Learning Environment

Overview

In the last chapter, we entered into a discussion on attention and effort in performance. Attention is an embodied,[1] self-regulatory system with many capabilities – focus, acuity, style, shift flexibility and more. Dancers learn to negotiate attention and effort by honing attention to movement dynamics. The honing of attention sharpens sense-ability,[2] a skill integral to attaining technical proficiency and artistic expressiveness. This chapter focuses on somatic learning as a unique context for training embodied attention. In Somatics, attending to sensory feedback is emphasized over movement choices or modes of execution. This learning context is reputed to help release bodily restrictions, discover new movement potential and promote autonomy. What remains to be discussed and debated is how somatic learning trains cognition. As dance researchers recontextualize embodied attention, Somatics stands to find a unique place within cognitive studies.

Focusing in…

- What is somatic learning?
- How does it compare to didactic- or other types of learning?
- What are the common elements in a somatic learning environment?
- How does this training environment differ from those of western dance?
- Describe the benefits of somatic learning.

Experiential prelude

Stop reading for a moment and get out a blank sheet of paper. Write down your name, your birth date and one task you have to do today…now pause. Repeat what you just wrote. Write the same sentences in the exact position (posture) you adopted previously – your facing, the angle of your body to the desk, paper and pen, the exact tempo in writing your sentences, the placement of your feet on the floor etc. Notice the challenge in trying to mimic yourself repeating the movement phrase exactly as you did before. Pause again…now write the phrase again attending to somatic information – your breathing, the feeling of your vitality, the pressure you exert on the pen, the texture of the paper *as* you write, the pressure you feel coming from the table and chair in their support of your arms and torso…and so forth. In the blink of an eye, you have shifted from a less conscious state of embodiment toward a more conscious enhanced one. Notice that the transformation didn't take much more than a shift in awareness and a refocusing of *attention*.[3] You shifted your attention toward the sensory information coming from bodily movement. These *somatic data* not only *in*form, but also *trans*form. They act dynamically, shifting your attention from the task itself to a more embodied state within the task. Somatic data abound. Paying attention to sensations arising from the body in stillness and movement provides a unique entry into embodied experience with distinctly different outcomes. How would you characterize this new state? Keep the experience in mind as you read the chapter.

Introduction

In several chapters, we've highlighted the contributions of cognitive neuroscientist Francisco Varela. Varela was pivotal in evolving a science of first-person consciousness. Earlier chapters recount Varela's work in evolving a science of lived experience (Varela 1996). To this end, Varela and his colleagues asked basic questions: What data can scientists gather from first person experience? How? What do these data tell us?

First-person data is ephemeral and elusive; at the same time, it is 'pragmatic' at its core (Varela and Shear 1999: 2). Sensible and practical, these data provide a *modus operandi* for making sense of the world. Varela wrote: first-person experience is 'pre-reflexive'…'a rich and largely unexplored source of information and data with dramatic consequences' (1999: 4). First-person experience is neither 'irreducible', nor 'derived from the third-person perspective' (1999: 3). Varela's pragmatism arose from his philosophical beliefs and meditative practices rooted in Buddhist and Vedic traditions. He supported many professional, pragmatic practices, including '…sports training, and psychotherapy' as 'privileged entry point for change (1999: 4–5). Varela was a scientist, not a movement artist or somatic practitioner. Thus, he also might have listed Somatics and dance or other movement studies among these practices.[4]

Today, scientists still struggle with validating first-person experience.[5] Even categorizing this kind of learning awaits a non-dualist paradigm. Today, the term that approximates an appropriate description of this type of learning is 'perceptuo-motor learning' (Buchanan and Ulrich 2001: 315). Here, sensory cues play a vital role in movement (motor) planning (Caeyenbergs et al. 2009). A few texts and studies lend support to an embodied cognitive approach to learning (Jeannerod 2006; Slepian et al. 2011; Moran et al. 2012). Limited evidence from neuro-imaging studies suggests that perceptuo-motor learning organizes brain networks. Imaging (brain-mapping) studies show a baseline of improved connectivity and communication between key regions of the cortex at rest (Khundrakpam et al. 2013; Lou, Joensson and Kringelbach 2011; Stawarczyk et al. 2011; van den Heuval and Hulshoff Pol 2010). Changes in the baseline modular organization of the brain resulting from perceptuo-motor learning suggest improved functional connectivity and efficiency (Yong et al. 2009). Although conjectural, interpretation of these brain maps suggests an enhanced mental state of readiness to respond and act (Stern et al. 2012).

This chapter returns to somatic learning methods as providing empirical data in support of embodied cognition. Somatic learning links body and mind through paying attention to sensory phenomena (often arising from movement – executed or imagined). A hallmark of Somatics lies in the method of learning to attend to sensory phenomena arising within a structured (movement) environment.

The compendium of *movement-based* somatic practices is diverse (Knaster 1993; Eddy 2009).[6] Commonalities of purpose and method exist, however. The learning environment usually affords the space and time to awaken embodied consciousness, focus attention, observe and hone sensory awareness and reflect on thoughts, feelings and actions. Learners attend to sensory information arising from: (1) their own movement and thoughts (improvised or prescriptive); (2) teacher-led, verbally guided lessons in sensory awareness/ attunement (through movement or stillness); (3) kinesthetic inter-subjectivity (the multi-layered experience of group learning contexts); and/or (4) the sensate qualities embedded within the environmental context. Focusing in these ways adds dimension and texture to embodied experience. Whether explicit goals are set or not, the process of sensing is more vital to the learning than movement choices or outcomes (Batson 1990). By sensitively honing attention to the cues or clues arising from the bodymind, the mover goes from simply becoming aware, to accessing deeper layers of experience.

Whether the environment is structured toward group- or self-exploration, there is ample opportunity to focus attention on sensory data. The somatic learning environment widens the intervals of time and space. Persons attend to sensory dynamics for a longer duration of time than they might ordinarily afford themselves in daily life. Practicing this *way* of attending builds self-regulatory skills. To paraphrase bodyworker Deanne Juhan (1987), if the mind (mentation) organizes the body for movement, the senses, in turn, organize the mind. Attending in this way shifts the learner away from the habitual embodiment status quo toward a deeper state of embodiment associated with greater movement potential and autonomy (Behnke 1997).

Somatic learning within dance

In the early decades of exposure to Somatics (roughly from the 1970s through the 1980s), dancers raised questions as to its fit within western contemporary dance pedagogy (Batson, Quin and Wilson 2012). In this period, somatic approaches emphasized slow, non-forceful movements. Much time was spent lying on the floor, out of gravity, paying attention to small sensory details or visual images in an atmosphere of non-doing. For this reason, somatic approaches were designated as non-techniques – therapeutic exercises rather than primary source material for artistic training (Green 2007; Batson 2008; Eddy 2009). Several decades of rich praxis interchange have changed this. Today, experimentation and growth in both domains have led to integrating Somatics into contemporary dance training (Fortin 1998; Bales and Nettl-Fiol 2008; Brodie and Lobel 2012). Somatic studies now are viewed as inroads to embodied knowing, basic to the ethics and ethos of dance education (Rouhiainen 2007; 2012): to developing a 'performative' and 'multiplicitous' bodily experience within dance (Hawksley 2011: 108), as well as to fostering movement creativity (Batson and Schwartz 2007; Rouhiainen 2012).

In dancemaking, movement-centered somatic learning is valued over other forms of didactic learning (Matthews 1998). This kind of learning also differs from mindfulness training, although positive outcomes have been reported from blending contemplative methods with choreography (Latitaraja 2012). Post-exploratory periods of reflection help dancers build a vocabulary for their own experience. These layers of experience are richly *cognitive*. They consist of 'reflective and discursive activity intended to facilitate the experiential flow between internal and external attention, implicit and explicit knowledge, intuitive and analytical states, perceptual and conceptual thought' (Clarke, Cramer and Müller 2010: 227).

Somatic movement experience disengages learners from 'the apprenticeship of observation' and mimicking, toward more autonomy in movement creation (Fortin 1998: 52). Experience of the somatic body fosters personal 'ownership and agency' (Hawksley 2011: 108),[7] and authority and empowerment (Eddy 2009; Green 2007; Green 1999; Fortin 1998). A guided somatic experience intends towards recognizing the body as a source of constructing knowledge while resisting claims made by dominant cultures (Gustafson 1999). These experiences encourage empathy and diversity through respecting and sharing experiential insights (Barlas 2001; Gustafson 1999).

Agent of change

How do somatic learning methods enact change?[8] In Somatics, honing sensitivity to bodily relationships is the starting place (Hanlon Johnson 2000: 479). Sensitivity arises out of basic human needs and desires – first and foremost, perhaps, being the need for safety. Sensitive attending is the change agent. In somatic learning, both ethos and agency lie in perceiving differences in bodily states. Attending to sensory data is not simply a matter of *noticing* these sensations; rather, the learning lies in noticing and registering *distinctions* and *differences* in the bodily status quo. To paraphrase scientist-futurist Gregory Bateson, true information is 'a difference that makes a difference' (Bateson (1978: 45). Perceivers become increasingly sensitive to sensory distinctions not detected in the tempo of everyday actions. Selectively attending to the senses reveals and registers experience. In daily life, people attend more readily to their tasks than themselves. In doing so, they are often displaced or alienated from lived embodiment (a phenomenon readers may have observed in the experiential prelude at the beginning of this chapter). Somatic learning transforms automatic habits of body obliviousness into enactive consciousness (Juhan 1987; Reeve 2011; Hanna 1970/1985).

Habits easily create a bodily profile that moves in ways that are conforming and obligatory. Awakening and attending to new sensations shift the compulsory toward new possibilities. Dynamic systems theory states that new coordination patterns emerge when habit is disturbed (Thelen and Smith 1994). To learn, habit needs a *perturbation* – a nudge to the body-context status quo. This nudge comes as a novel stimulus to the brain. It awakens and enlivens neural processes, enabling plasticity and learning. Perturbations move the perceiver away from the familiar toward new possibilities for action.

The implications for dancers are multifold. In dance, the moving self *is* the task. If habitual movement patterns set in, they may limit movement potential and/or mask our limitations (Behnke 1997). Such limitations not only close the door to new, fresh experiences, but also may lead to dysfunction and injury (Hanna 1970/1985). Somatic learning 'reveals tendencies towards fixity in the patterns that characterize the bodyscape' (Hawksley 2011: 108). Through a process of embodied differentiation and discernment, movement skill emerges. Here, listening to and reflecting on somatic experience deepens embodied knowledge and promotes movement efficiency (Clarke, Kramer and Müller 2010).

Further, newly embodied states foster autonomy and feed the creative process (Kampe 2010; Long, Warwick and Fortin 2012). Emphasis lies in the process of developing a lively 'tension between facilitating the development of specificity and control in decision-making and embracing freedom and difference of response…more emphasis is on the "making it one's own," on individual choice and decision-making within the performance of the material – less on a preoccupation with memorization…Skills of attention, imagination and curiosity are "thought through" the body to become tools of…physical proficiency' (Clarke, Cramer and Müller 2010: 223). Further, attention technique builds from both individual and collaborative processes 'that are reflective, self-generative, and socially-inclusive practice… [processes bridging across] dance, health and education' (Kampe 2010: 34).

Essential ingredients

While each somatic method structures its training environment uniquely, common elements exist. Constraints[9] on the learning environment include:

1. Providing an atmosphere free of judgment (Kaparo 2012)

The learner should enter a place that feels safe and not push himself/herself – or be pushed – to learn. This atmosphere helps set the stage for training the focus of attention to honing sensitivity. The somatic learning environment affords a unique space and place for honing sensory *acuity*. The atmosphere is one of relative *non-doing*, meaning, instructions are directed toward discovery, rather than goal attainment. An atmosphere of curiosity and playful exploration replaces trying hard to achieve movement goals (Clarke, Kramer and Müller 2010; Batson and Schwartz 2007). Sensing, not imposing preconceived notions or thoughts about what should happen, allows the inner narrative, the levels of implicit knowing, to surface more readily. The emphasis is on the process (*how* to do the movement) rather than the outcome (what the movement is expected to become) (Stinson 1995; Batson 1990). By honoring the present moment of learning, the dancer is more readily open to an experience of 'somatic disclosure', a means of accessing the deeper self – embodied and unified (Lowman, Jourard and Jourard 1994).

2. Sensory privileging (Green 2002)

The somatic learning environment prefaces or 'privileges' (Green 2002: 114), sensory information coming from the body. Attending to sensory information is a unique way of mining bodily data. The intent usually is different from that of meditation, where mental (tacit) messages are repeated explicitly to quiet the mind. Rather, learners move, attending to exploring a range of sensory qualities (qualia) depending on instruction: visual, auditory, somato-sensory, vestibular and many other unnamed senses. The focus of attention on movement dynamics can be either in a feed-forward or feedback manner. *Feed-forward* means before the fact – in other words, imagining an action before performing it to prime the neurons needed to execute the movement. *Feedback* means after the fact – attending to the sensations arising from movement. In either case, the learner prolongs the interval of attending and tracks and/or guides emergent sensory data. Focused attention also gives rise to a wealth of vague sensations. These are preverbal, prenoetic sensations; for example, they might be 'the feeling of what happens' (Damasio 1999) or the 'felt sense' (Gendlin 1992: 203). The body infers more than can be construed through verbal concepts or distinctions. Such disclosure provides an intricacy and intimacy of experience evaded by everyday language (Gendlin 1992).

3. Augmenting rest (Batson and Schwartz 2007)

An atmosphere of non-doing is one of augmented rest. Somatic learning embeds resting phases into movement exploration or visualization practices. The resting phase usually is at least as long as the activity phase (Batson and Schwartz 2007; Batson 2009). A class often involves a 'physical component' or 'charge', in which the body is stimulated to move from its current state, followed by some time interval of open attention in reflection (Clarke, Cramer and Müller 2010: 223). A 'moving phase' is counterbalanced by a 'resting phase' (Batson 2009). In the resting phase, two things can happen: (1) the learner lets go of attending or moving and just rests; and (2) the learner stops moving or priming thinking (the 'charge') and just listens to the sensory feedback arising from movement or other internal cues. The feedback is likened to throwing a pebble in a lake or to striking one note on a piano. The harmonics of this one 'charge' keep playing out for a long time. This is the opposite of what often is stressed in physical training, where rest is not as valued as repetition. Motor-learning research refers to this kind of activity-to-rest ratio as distributed practice (Batson 2009; Batson and Schwartz 2007; Schmidt and Lee 1988).

Neurologically, the resting phase is a time for attention to go *off-line*. When ample time is given for resting and reflecting, the expanded interval affords the nervous system the time to make sense of inner sensations and signals that are integral to self-organization, proprioceptive guidance and control. Going slowly and paying attention to the events within the various phases of movement, the nervous system is given time for processing and integration. The resting interval impacts on the strength of many cognitive faculties (Yang, Gallo and Beilock 2009). Rest improves memory consolidation, recall and actual performance (Batson 2009 for review). When rest is afforded equal status to practice, the bodymind is refreshed and new learning readily surfaces. Habitual attitudes and behaviors are less likely to reoccur in the face of rested presence. The resting interval can be very brief (Alexander Technique's pausing and inhibiting), brief (the typical two-to-three minute rest between repetition and variation in Feldenkrais Awareness Through Movement), fairly long (20 minutes or more of Ideokinetic Constructive Rest) or longer (a full night's sleep or an extended retreat, for example).

In summary, attention is attuned in Somatics to distinguishing differences in sensory dynamics in expanded space-time. The somatic learning environment within dancemaking may or may not be constructed differently from the actual dance context. The importance in cultivating embodied knowledge lies in gaining an understanding of the interrelationship between attention and effort. The type of attention … and the letting go of attending – all these phases are important in learning effortless control. Today, many approaches have bridged between early Somatic practices and contemporary dance, Skinner Release Technique (and other release techniques) among them (Emslie 2009). Several approaches have been codified in the dance classroom (Fortin, Vieria and Tremblay 2009), and many new dance forms have emerged which blur the edges between the two fields. The next two chapters describe two somatic approaches as cases for the effectiveness of somatic methods in training attention.

'Questions forward' for Chapter 7 appear in Appendix II.

References

Alexander, F.M. (1932/2001), *The Use of the Self*, London: Orion Books, Ltd.

Barlas, C. (2001), 'Learning-within-relationship as context and process in adult education' in R.O. Smith et al. (eds.), 42nd Annual Adult Education Research Conference Proceedings, East Lansing, Michigan, 1–3 June 2001.

Bales, M. and Nettl-Fiol, R. (eds.) (2008), *The Body Eclectic: Evolving Practices in Dance Training*, Urbana and Chicago: University of Illinois Press.

Bateson, G. (1978), 'Number is different from quantity', *CoEvolution Quarterly*, Spring, pp. 44–46.

Batson, G. (1990), 'Dancing fully, safely and expressively: The role of the body therapies in dance training', *Journal of Physical Education, Recreation and Dance*, 61: 9, pp. 28–31.

—— (2008), 'Teaching alignment', in M. Bales and R. Nettl-Fiol (eds.), *The Body Eclectic: Evolving Practices in Dance Training*. Urbana and Chicago: University of Illinois Press, pp. 134–52.

—— (2009), 'The somatic practice of intentional rest in dance education: Preliminary steps towards a method of study', *Journal of Dance and Somatic Practices*, 1: 2, pp. 177–97.

—— and Schwartz, R.E. (2007), 'Revisiting the value of somatic education in dance training through an inquiry into practice schedules', *Journal of Dance Education*, 7: 2, pp. 47–56.

——, Wilson, M. and Quin, E. (2012), 'Integrating somatics and science', *Journal of Dance and Somatic Practices*, 3: 1–2, pp. 183–93.

Behnke, E. (1997), 'Ghost gestures: Phenomenological investigations of bodily micromovements and their intercorporeal implications', *Human Studies*, 20: 2, pp. 181–201.

Brodie, J.A. and Lobel, E.E. (2012), *Dance and Somatics: Mind-Body Principles of Teaching and Performance*, Jefferson, NC: McFarland & Company, Inc.

Buchanan, P.A. and Ulrich, B.D. (2001), 'The Feldenkrais Method: A dynamic approach to changing motor behavior', *Research Quarterly for Exercise and Sport*, 72: 4, pp. 315–23.

Caeyenberghs, K., Wilson, P.H., van Roon, D., Swinnen, S.P. and Smits-Engelsman, C.M. (2009), 'Increasing convergence between imagined and executed movements across development: Evidence for the emergence of movement representations', *Developmental Science*, 12, pp. 474–83.

Clarke, G., Cramer, F. and Müller, G. (2010), 'Minding motion' in I. Diehl and F. Lampert (eds.), *Dance Techniques 2010*, Leipzig: Henschel Verlag, pp. 199–229.

Damasio, A. (1999), *The Feeling of What Happens*, New York, NY: Harcourt.

Eddy, M. (2009), 'A brief history of somatic practices and dance: Historical development of the field of somatic education and its relationship to dance', *Journal of Dance and Somatic Practices*, 1: 1, pp. 5–27.

Emslie, M. (2009), 'Skinner Releasing Technique: Dancing from within', *Journal of Dance and Somatic Practices*, 1: 2, pp. 169–75.

Feldenkrais, M. (1981), *The Elusive Obvious*, Cupertino, CA: Meta Publications.

Fortin, S. (1998), 'Somatics: A Tool for Empowering Modern Dance Teachers' in S.B. Shapiro (ed.), *Dance, Power, and Difference: Critical and Feminist Perspectives on Dance Education*, Champaign, IL: Human Kinetics, pp. 49–74.

Fortin, S., Vieria, A. and Tremblay, M. (2009), 'The experience of discourses in dance and somatics', *Journal of Dance and Somatic Practices*, 1: 1, pp. 47–64.

Gallagher, S. (2006), *How the Body Shapes the Mind*, New York, NY: Oxford University Press.

Gendlin, E. (1992), 'The wider role of bodily sense in thought and language' in M. Sheets-Johnstone (ed.), *Giving the Body its Due*, Albany, NY: State University of New York Press, pp. 192–207.

Green, J. (1999), 'Somatic authority and the myth of the ideal body in dance education', *Dance Research Journal*, 31: 2, pp. 80–100.

—— (2002), 'Somatic knowledge: The body as content and methodology in dance education', *Journal of Dance Education*, 2, pp. 113–18.

——— (2007), 'Student bodies: Dance pedagogy and the Soma', *International Handbook of Research in Arts Education*, pp. 1119–35.

Gustafson, D.L. (1999), 'Embodied learning: The body as an epistemological site' in M. Mayberry and E.C. Rose (eds.), *Meeting the Challenge: Innovative Feminist Pedagogies in Action*, New York, NY: Routledge, pp. 249–74.

Hanna, T. (1970/1985), *Bodies in Revolt: A Primer in Somatic Thinking*, New York, NY Reinhart and Winston.

Hanlon Johnson, D. (2000), 'Intricate tactile sensitivity: A key variable in western integrative bodywork', *Progress in Brain Research*, 122, pp. 479–90. http://donhanlonjohnson.com/articles/intricate.html. Accessed 12 February 2013.

Hawksley, S. (2011), 'Choreographic and somatic strategies for navigating bodyscapes and tensegrity schemata', *Journal of Dance & Somatic Practices*, 3: 1–2, pp. 101–10.

Jeannerod, M. (2006), *Motor Cognition: What Actions Tell the Self*, New York, NY: Oxford University Press.

Juhan, D. (1987), *Job's Body: A Handbook for Bodyworkers*, Barrytown, NY: Stationhill Press.

Kampe, T. (2010), '"Weave": The Feldenkrais Method as choreographic process', *Performio*, 1: 2, pp. 34–52.

Kaparo, R.F. (2012), *Awakening Somatic Intelligence: The Art and Practice of Embodied Mindfulness*, Berkeley, CA: North Atlantic Books.

Khundrakpam, B.S., Reid, A. and Brauer, J. et al. (2013), 'Developmental changes in organization of structural brain networks', *Cerebral Cortex*, 23: 9, pp. 2072–85.

Knaster, M. (1993), *Discovering the Body's Wisdom*, New York, NY: Bantam Books.

Lalitaraja, J.C. (2012), 'A Buddhist's approach to choreography as spiritual practice', *Journal of Dance and Somatic Practices*, 4: 1, pp. 143–54.

Long, Warwick and Fortin, S. (2012), *Integrating the Feldenkrais Method Within the Dance Classroom*, http://ebookbrowse.com/warwick-long-sylvie-fortin-dance-pdf-d361919073. Accessed 20 January 2013.

Lou, H.C., Joensson, M. and Kringelbach, M.L. (2011), 'Yoga lessons for consciousness research: A paralimbic network balancing brain resource allocation', *Frontiers in Psychology*, 2, pp. 366–72.

Lowman, M., Jourard, A. and Jourard, M. (eds.) (1994), *Sidney Jourard: Collected Writings*, Berkeley, CA: Round Right Press.

Matthews, J.C. (1998), 'Somatic knowing and education', *Educational Forum*, 62: 3, pp. 236–42.

Moran, A., Guillot, A., MacIntyre, T. and Collet, C. (2012), 'Re-imagining motor imagery: Building bridges between cognitive neuroscience and sport psychology', *British Journal of Psychology*, 103, pp. 224–47.

Petitmengin, C. (ed.) (2009), *Ten Years of Viewing From Within: The Legacy of Francisco Varela*, Exeter, UK: Imprint Academic.

Reeve, S. (2011), *Nine Ways of Seeing the Body*, Axminster, UK: Triarchy Press.

Rouhiainen, L. (ed.) (2007), *Ways of Knowing in Dance and Art*, *Acta Scenica*, 19, Helsinki: Helsinki Theatre Academy.

Rouhiainen, L. (2012), 'An investigation into facilitating the work of the independent contemporary dancer through somatic psychology', *Journal of Dance and Somatic Practices*, 3: 1–2, pp. 43–59.

Schmidt, R.A. and Lee, T. (1988), *Motor Control and Learning: A Behavioral Emphasis*, Champaign, IL: Human Kinetics Press.

Sheets-Johnstone, M. (2011), *The Primacy of Movement*, 2nd edn, Charlottesville, VA: John Benjamin Publisher.

Slepian, M.L., Weisbuch, M., Rule, N.O. and Ambady, N. (2011), 'Tough and tender: Embodied categorization of gender', *Psychological Science*, 22, pp. 26–28.

Stawarczyk, D., Majerus, D., Maquet, P. and D'Argembeau, A. (2011), 'Neural correlates of ongoing conscious experience: Both task-unrelatedness and stimulus-independence are related to default network activity', *PLoS ONE*, http://www.plosone.org/article/info:doi/10.1371/journal.pone.0016997. Accessed 13 February 2013.

Stern, E.R., Fitzgerald, K.D., Welsh, R.C., Abelson, J.L. and Taylor, S.F. (2012), 'Resting-state functional connectivity between fronto-parietal and default mode networks in obsessive-compulsive disorders', *PLoS ONE*, http://www.plosone.org/article/info:doi/10.1371/journal.pone.0036356. Accessed 12 February 2013.

Stinson, S.W. (1995), 'Body of knowledge', *Educational Theory*, 45: 1, pp. 43–54.

Thelen and Smith 1994), *Dynamic Systems Approach to the Development of Cognition and Action*. Cambridge, MA: The MIT Press.

Thompson, E. (ed.) (2001), *Between Ourselves: Second Person Issues in the Study of Consciousness*, Thorverton, UK: Imprint Academic, 2001. Published simultaneously as a special triple issue of the *Journal of Consciousness Studies* 8: 5–7.

van den Heuval, M.P. and Hulshoff Pol, H.E. (2010), 'Exploring the brain network: A review on resting-state fMRI functional connectivity', *European Neuropsychopharmacology*, 20: 8, pp. 519–34.

Varela, F. (1996), 'Neurophenomenology: A methodological remedy for the hard problem', *Journal of Consciousness Studies*, 3: 4, pp. 330–49.

Varela, F.J. and Shear, J. (1999), 'First person methodologies: What, why, how?', *Journal of Consciousness Studies*, 6: 2–3, pp. 1–14.

Yang, S., Gallo, D. and Beilock, S.L. (2009), 'Embodied memory judgments: A case of motor fluency', *Journal of Experiment Psychology: Learning, Memory, & Cognition*, 35, pp. 1359–65.

Yong, H., Wang, J., Wang, L. et al. (2009), 'Uncovering intrinsic modular organization of spontaneous brain activity in humans', *PLoS ONE*, http://www.plosone.org/article/info%3Adoi%2F10.1371%2Fjournal.pone.0005226. Accessed 11 February 2013.

Notes

1   Here, the term 'embodiment' means the general sense of mind-body unity, also called 'psychophysical unity' (Alexander 1932). One of the earliest uses of this term in the Somatic literature appeared in F.M. Alexander's book, *The Use of the Self* (1932/2001) to connote agency, rather than just mental states or states of sensory awareness.

2　The term 'sense-ability' is adapted from *SenseAbility* – a newsletter of applications of the Feldenkrais Method. For an example of this newsletter, see Galeota-Wozny (2001), issue 21, http://www.feldenkrais.com/download/senseability/sense21.pdf.

3　Movement educator Moshe Feldenkrais referred to this phenomenon as 'the elusive obvious', as reflected in his book of the same name (Feldenkrais 1981).

4　Adding the pragmatic method was pivotal to advancing a first-person methodology in science, and yet has been critiqued as not going far enough. See Sheets-Johnstone (2011).

5　The dearth of scientific studies on somatic learning in part lies in the same challenges Varela faced in forging a model for embodiment science (subjective and inter-subjective). Somatics and dance continue to be underrepresented in embodied cognitive theory. For recent reviews on this challenge, see Petitmengin (2009) and Thompson (2001).

6　Somatic education falls roughly into two categories – active, consciously aware, movement-based practices and more practices where the learner is more quiet and receptive (massage, cranio-sacral therapy etc.). In this book, we emphasize the former as more readily integrated into dance settings.

7　These terms 'ownership and agency' are associated with the work of cognitive phenomenologist, Shaun Gallagher. Gallagher uses these terms to explain two brain phenomena: body image and body schema. His work is pivotal in investigating the brain–body connection. Through studying sensory deafferentation and other neurological forms of sensory loss, Gallagher outlined neurological concepts of having a body (ownership) and acting from the body (agency). See Gallagher (2006). Here, Sue Hawksley uses the terms to explain aspects of bodily empowerment.

8　A change agent can take many forms. Different somatic practices afford unique opportunities. For example, a dancer experiencing an Alexander Technique lesson might attune to the experience of rapid, reflex reactions of postural synergies when given a verbal cue to rise from a chair. Another dancer in a Feldenkrais Awareness Through Movement lesson might attune to global changes in muscle tone, by attending to the movement feedback. Here, movements are performed in small range, 'effortlessly' (i.e., performed below the level of muscular effort associated with goal achievement). A third dancer might explore the various qualities underscoring the concept of *mind* of the tissue, common to Body-Mind Centering exercises.

9　See Chapter 3 for further explanation of tasks and constraints.

Chapter 8

Somatic Approaches to Training Attention: Part I
The Mental Practice of Motor Imagery

Cognition is 'a dynamic process of knowing'.

(Thinus-Blanc and Gaunet 1999: 294)

Overview

Visualizing imagery is a unique cognitive process. Visualizing movement primes the motor centers in the brain, activating the neurons designated for the intended movement. Dancers can look back to nearly a century of visualization practice called Ideokinesis. This practice dated from the 1930s, in the work of Mabel Todd and later, Todd's student, Lulu Sweigard. Ideokinesis initially was designed to re-educate faulty mechanical alignment through visualizing motor imagery. Sweigard devised the 'constructive rest position', a position of mechanical advantage where dancers activate their imagination and attend to anatomical detail while resting their bodies. For over a century, as well, sports and exercise science subscribed to a method similar to Ideokinesis – *mental rehearsal* or *mental practice*. Here, athletes watch (imagine) themselves performing skilled movement sequences within their sport-specific contexts. With the advent of imaging methods in neuroscience, the term *mental practice of motor imagery* (MPMI) (Jackson et al. 2001) gained popularity as an effective method for rehabilitating the physical dysfunctions caused by neurological disorders such as stroke (Decety 1996a; 1996b; Jeannerod 1997). More than a third of a century of scientific evidence from imaging studies now supports the use of mental practice for neuromuscular re-education. At the same time, many issues continue to challenge the theory that visualizing an action is neurologically equivalent to performing it. This chapter provides an update on the contemporary models of MPMI. As a prime example of embodied cognition, MPMI remains a useful tool for improving motor skills.

Focusing in…

- How would you define *motor* imagery from other forms of imagery?
- Describe how imagining an action actually differs from performing it.
- How has mental practice benefited your dance experience (or not)?

- What factors would be important to consider in designing dance research involving mental practice of motor imagery?

Experiential prelude

Sit quietly, keeping your eyes open. Imagine yourself steadily *running* somewhere – it doesn't matter what context – a city street, a grassy lane, a beach. See yourself clearly for about 20 seconds. Be aware of the kinesthetic (feeling) state of this action while you picture yourself as clearly as possible in your imagination. Now keep this image of *running* in your mind and say out loud the word *throwing*. How easy is it to do one activity in your mind while your speech muscles *execute* another? Perhaps you experienced a little cognitive dissonance? Try the same experiment with your eyes closed. This exercise reveals the power of the brain's motor drive. It is nearly impossible to visualize one action clearly while trying to perform two actions. Focusing your attention on one action absorbs the bulk of this limited resource, leaving little capacity for multitasking.

Introduction

Since ancient times mental imagery has been a vital source for understanding experience (Samuels and Samuels 1975). Visualization is one way our bodymind both 'represents' and 'simulates' reality.[1] Mentally engaging the *mind's eye* acts as a kind of mental bridge, providing a pathway from the possible to the probable. Considered integral to the health of human consciousness, mental imagery takes form through many different sensory modalities – visual, auditory, tactile-kinesthetic, olfactory and nebulous, unnamed synaesthetic experiences (Kosslyn, Thompson and Ganis 2006). Emerging in infancy, images help the developing child in ways that are pre-propositional, pre-linguistic, and embodied (Sheets-Johnstone 2010). Throughout life, this kind of embodied thinking affords humans many ways of understanding and acting intelligently in the world (Johnson 1998).

Since the turn of the twentieth century, scientists suspected that merely thinking of movement activated the same motor portions of the brain. Neuroscientist William Benjamin Carpenter called this phenomenon 'the ideomotor principle' (Carpenter 1852: 148). The twentieth century saw the extended use of motor imagery in sports and (later) in dance. Mental imagery practice for improvement of motor performance became the focus of rigorous research in sports psychology (Feltz and Landers 1983; Murphy and Martin 2002; Pearson et al. 2013) and neuroscience (Mulder 2007; McNorgan 2012). Primary benefits include enhancing physical performance and developing cognitive and coping skills in elite sports competitions (e.g., skill acquisition, confidence and relaxation techniques). In rehabilitation medicine, mental imagery practice is used for recovery and re-education of physical skills (Jackson et al. 2001; Dickstein and Deutsch 2007; Batson 2004).

In dance, several generations of dancers benefited from the works of the early pioneers who taught and wrote eloquently on this living anatomical science.[2] Dance practitioners published guides to practice (Dowd 1995; Franklin 1996; 2012; Krasnow and Deveau 2010). Over the last decade, a number of dance-specific reviews on imagery have surfaced (Nordin and Cumming 2005; 2007; Murphy, Nordin and Cumming 2008); others report psychophysical or technical benefits (e.g., Jola, Angharad and Haggard 2011; Goldschmidt 2002; Coker et al. 2012). The effects of different modes of visual imagery on choreography and movement creation also have been examined (e.g., de LaHunta and Barnard 2005; May et al. 2011). Further, the empirical window on imagery research in dance recently has broadened with the addition of imaging technology (May et al. 2011).

Despite robust reviews, rigorous research designs remain difficult to locate, however. Models for mental practice of *motor* imagery (Jackson et al. 2001) did not gain scientific credibility until the 1980s (Guillot et al. 2012). The psychometric values of visualization are not easy to measure using any behavioral battery or imaging technology (Kosslyn Thompson and Ganis 2006). Intrinsic (personal) and interpersonal differences influence the nature of the image itself, its usage and outcomes (Holmes and Calmels 2008; Moran et al. 2012). Extrinsic variables also play a role. Thinking *while* moving and thinking *about* movement are fundamentally tied to person and context. Below, we revisit the topic of motor imagery, with the intent to clarify key concepts relevant to designing dance imagery research.

Motor imagery practice – definition and function

A working definition of the MPMI comes from several sources from sports and exercise science and cognitive neuroscience. MPMI is '...the neural generation or regeneration of parts of a brain representation/neural network involving primarily top-down sensorial, perceptual and affective characteristics, that are primarily under the conscious control of the imager and which may occur in the absence of perceptual afference functionally equivalent to the actual sporting experience' (Morris et al. 2005: 14). MPMI also is described as 'a dynamic mental state during which the representation of a given motor act or movement is rehearsed in working memory without any overt motor output' (Guillot and Collet 2008: 31). In other words, the practitioner assumes a relaxed state, without actually moving or exerting any effort by intending to move (Jeannerod 2006).[3] During mental practice, it is essential that no voluntary muscular force (contraction) be added during the visualization process (Sweigard 1974). Accurate neural programming of an action depends on how clearly the goal is visualized (Granit 1980). The goal incorporates the speed, trajectory and dynamics of the image, although the imager may not actually experience these dynamics fully.

For athletics and dance, MPMI is an exercise in motor learning. It is a key way of training embodied attention; that is, training the focus of attention to refining the details related to optimizing skilled physical performance (Murphy, Nordin and Cumming 2008).

Mental practice for motor performance enhancement is designed to support the health of the neuromuscular system by:

1.   uncovering habitual patterns of effort that interfere with optimal performance;
2.   redirecting maladaptive patterns toward improved movement freedom and expertise;
3.   learning new patterns of movement without undue mental or physical effort; and
4.   memorizing, rehearsing, and/or perfecting movement without the added physiological and cognitive burden of actual execution (Murphy, Nordin and Cumming 2008).

In MPMI, people mentally rehearse (visualize) an action while simultaneously suppressing any attempt to perform the action. To be classified as *motor* imagery, the image must move. The image ideally contains the same kinetics (force dynamics) as the actual movement itself. Picturing an apple, for example, does not necessarily convey a sense of movement. Nonetheless, a picture of an apple can contain aspects of *motricity* – the smell of a rose, for example, evokes memories full of animated qualities – the speed, direction, spatial expansion, degree of intensity, degree of kinesthetic absorption, affective mood and other kinesthetic and kinetic aspects of movement certainly are captured in the experience.

These dynamic attributes of the motor image are agents of change.[4] Mental practice stimulates change in a feed-forward way. The cognitive process of mentally visualizing movement causes neural activation of the same movement, albeit at a lower level of activation than actual performance. According to neuroscientist Marc Jeannerod, mentally imagining action is not only a 'representation' of an action, but also an actual 'simulation' of motor action (2006: 24, 27). Persons observing the action are actually *doing* the action. At the same time, they are programming the brain to learn aspects of the action. The MPMI shares similar neurological substrates with those involved in actual execution of the action (Decety 1996a). Neurological substrates in this case suggest similar synaptic patterns and network connectivity. This implies that MPMI might follow the same biomechanical and functional rules that govern actual execution of goal-directed actions.[5]

This suggests that mental practice is not solely a mental act, but a somatic act of bodymind holism. Some argue that motor imagery is not an abstract 'mental "picture," "construct," or "schema"…[as] these have no basis in experience and are best a type of explanatory convenience, a hypothetical entity in the brain…that is conjured to do the work of putting movement together, furnishing a kinetic blueprint for the neurological eyes only…' (Sheets-Johnstone 2009: 269–70). Images, schemas and constructs fail to capture the dynamics of movement – whether imagined or executed. Movement experience generates neural imagery rather than the other way around. Being able to conjure up an image of motor action is possible because the person remembers the experience of actually doing this action. Because the motor image contains within it the kinematic and kinetic *qualia* of a movement experience to some degree.

Mentally practicing motor imagery is not one undifferentiated cognitive faculty or event. The imager visualizes an action and experiences its somatic effects before, during and after the visualization period. Imagers also can visualize movement from multiple vantage points. From these different phenomenological vantage points imagers either can immerse themselves in an experience, or distance themselves from experience. For example, you either can experience being present in an activity, or watch yourself from a distance (watching your own movie). Although some might argue that both states are possible simultaneously (Depraz, Varela and Vermersch 2003), scientists distinguish these two vantage points as distinct neural phenomena. Neurologically, the frame of reference is coded in the nervous system differently and labeled as *egocentric* or *allocentric* (Decety 1996a; Jeannerod 1997). Each vantage point offers a distinct sensory experience and activates different brain processes (Jeannerod 2006; Clark et al. 2003). Analyzing the effects of MPMI requires speculating on the neural substrates from these two separate vantage points (Decety 1996a; 1996b). Defining the vantage point for visualizing, therefore, is essential in research designs.

As mentioned, the MPMI obeys motor rules and biomechanical constraints to a certain extent. For example, MPMI follows Fitt's law (speed-accuracy trade-off) (Jeannerod 2006: 132). The faster one tries to either execute or mentally imagine an action, the more muddy the details of execution. Imagined action also exhibits *isosynchrony*. Isosynchrony means that the time frame for execution of motor imagery is equivalent to that of actual physical execution (Calmels et al. 2006; Decety, Jeannerod and Prablanc 1989; Guillot and Collet 2005). The more physically complex the movement task, the longer the duration of mental time to achieve it (Georgopoulos and Massey 1987). Whether or not greater efficiency can be trained is conjectural. MPMI also obeys similar rules governing joint kinematics and degrees of freedom (Jeannerod 2006: 132). As tasks increase in complexity, imagining the entire sequence with clarity becomes increasingly difficult. This is a common phenomenon in dance when trying to recall and execute an intricate movement phrase.

At the same time, a motor image is not the exact same neural process as actual physical execution. This is because: (1) the neural activation is weaker; (2) the activation is coupled with suppression (inhibition) of motor output – a prerequisite for off-line representation of the action; and (3) the muscles do not actually contract (and the body does not move). Thus, sensory feedback normally accompanying full-out movement execution is lacking (Jeannerod 2006).

This is an important factor in physical training. In motor imagery practice, 'one experiences the bodily sensations of movement, not the movement commands themselves' (Moulton and Kosslyn 2009: 1273). Physical practice is a must, therefore, regardless of how precisely the mental image is practiced. Without physical practice, it is difficult to experience the range of force dynamics intrinsic to the action through imagination alone (Jeannerod 2006). While a sampling of research supports the concept that mental practice alone can improve skilled sports performance, the weight of the evidence states that physical practice is necessary for motor-skill learning. At the same time, however, motor-skill learning is enhanced when mental practice and physical practice are combined (i.e., stronger motor learning effects than when either is done alone) (Feltz and Landers 1983; Feltz, Landers and Becker 1988; Murphy and Martin 2002).

Coordinated imagined action also can emerge from a task context. For example, researchers in two different studies examined the type of grip needed to grasp a dowel orientated at eight different angles in a computerized display. Participants were asked to choose a grip that would minimize postural discomfort and maximize efficiency. In most cases, the participants visualized and selected the appropriate grasp (Rosenbaum et al. 2004; Johnson 2000). In this case, task constraints organized the movement. This resonates with Sheets-Johnstone's perspective on 'schemas' (noted above). Sheets-Johnstone speculates that no image or schema stands between the mover and the object to be moved. Other studies bear this out, as well. Recognizing the appropriate hand (right or left) in pictures of rotated hands, suggests the action is primarily a motor task – rather than a visual imagery task. While these results here are compelling, gaining a sense of the whole body in its task context remains a research challenge (Jola, Angharad and Haggard 2009).

In the end, it appears that motor imagery is a much more complex act than previously thought. More likely, motor imagery practice involves 'two separate sets of cognitive skills' (Moran et al. 2012: 237): 'a true mental simulation of the real action, and a more creative process that could include manipulating the visual representation of the action, making inferences based on non-motor cues, or retrieving motor memories' (Deprati et al. 2010: 1028). Despite discrepancies in research, there appear to be overall general benefits from the use of MPMI that outweigh the difficulties. These include:

1. Portability – mental imagery can be practiced almost anywhere;
2. Effort reduction – mental practice is dissociated from actual physical practice, thereby minimizing physical and mental fatigue, particularly in high-pressured situations of competition and performance; and
3. Neural priming – mental practice activates the same neuron pools as those involved in performing the task, but to a much smaller degree (Hugdahl 2009). Thus, mental practice of motor imagery stimulates motor-skill learning, but skill improvement requires physical practice.

Challenges remaining

To date, preliminary findings are promising on training attention (focusing the mind) through mental imagery practice (Driskell et al. 1994; Lutz et al. 2008; Travis and Shear 2010). Research is needed to test the effectiveness of training that links visual attention to motor learning. For example, while MPMI still is used extensively within dance with expressed benefits for improving alignment (Krasnow and Deveau 2010), its effects on posture remain controversial (deLange, Helmich and Toni 2006).

Our understanding and use of imagery research is hampered by a number of challenges: '[l]ack of consistency in definitions, descriptions of imagery, and protocols' (Morris et al 2005: 14), and reporting of instructions and demonstration. Explicit instructions and practice conditions rarely are outlined or reported in any published literature (Magali et al. 2008; McCullagh and Weiss 2001; Krasnow and Deveau 2010).

Second, research on motor imagery is influenced by many factors that impact on success of the outcomes: the population and purpose of the imagery being studied, the level of the imager's experience, the degree of familiarity with the task and whether the task has been memorized in advance of the testing or not, the participant's general ability to visualize actions in relation to the limitations of imaging batteries (Calmels et al. 2006). Different populations require specific goals for mental practice. For example, a protocol might be designed to help a young adolescent female dancer gain increased staccato dynamics (increased 'spring') when rising on pointe. A very different protocol would be needed to address the needs of a more seasoned female dancer (age 40, for example), who needs to enhance the health of musculo-tendinous tissue of her calves to improve the preparation before a jump (see Table 8.1 for ideas for designing imagery protocols for specific dance populations).

Important directions for research lie in investigating meta-imagery processes – that is, people's knowledge of their own mental imagery skills and sense of control over their imagery experience (Moran et al. 2012: 238; Moran 2009; MacIntyre and Moran 2010). Behavioral methods of measuring imagery have multiple challenges (Nordin and Cumming 2007; Calmels et al. 2006). Questions still arise as to what is being measured – vividness, clarity, degree of absorption or other psychometric factors – and other critical questions continue to be raised (see Box 8.1). Dance researchers are poised to take these questions to the next level.

Table 8.1: Guidelines for mental practice protocols for diverse dance populations

Who?	Age	Suggested purpose or goal	Body focus – vantage point	Qualitative outcomes	Quantitative outcome(s)[1] 'effect'
Novice	11	Enhance turn-out	Hip joint – internal	Static & dynamic alignment	Measurable increase range of motion – attainment of joint neutral
Intermediate student	18	Increase depth of plié in initial phase of jumping	Lower limb joints – Internal to external	Efficient mechanics to decrease fatigue	Measurable increase in jump height – efficient use of ground reaction forces – motion analysis
New company member	24	Improve gestural line of the arm	Head-neck, upper quarter joints – internal to external	Detecting and correcting aesthetic errors	Explicit improvements in timing & sequencing – motion analysis
Elite dance artist	33	Increase variability & range of a diagonal reach of the arms	Upper-to-lower trunk relationships – internal to external	Whole body connection/expression	Increased spatial dynamics, decreased timing – motion analysis
Dance educator	44	Restore full range post-injury muscle strain to the calf (gastrocnemius)	Dorsiflexors – internal	Greater extensibility without compensation	Measurable improvement in ankle-foot range of motion and tissue quality
Performance artist	64	Improve poised balance in a lateral weight shift	Dynamic lumbo-pelvic mobility – internal to external	Smoother transitions between movements without errors	Reduced number of errors (e.g., wobbling, near falls)
Retired mentor	82	Enhance sensory sensitivity to decrease compressive forces in weight bearing	Femoral bone tissue internal	Enhanced kinesthetic sensitivity and sense of mobility in micro-movements	Measurable decrease in fall risk and improvement in tissue quality – imaging studies

[1] Neuro-imaging and other quantitative measures often conducted by physical rehabilitation specialists

Adapted from: Munroe, J.J., Giacobbi, P.R., Hall, C., and Weinberg, R. (2000), 'The four W's of imagery use: where, when, why, and what?', *The Sport Psychologist*, 14, pp. 119–37; Holmes, P.S. and Collins, D.J. (2001), 'The PETTLEP approach to motor imagery: A functional equivalence model for sport psychologists', *Journal of Applied Sport Psychology*, 13, pp. 60–83. This seven-element model outlines the physical, environment, task, timing, learning, emotion and perspective aspects of imagery protocols.

Box 8.1: A sampling of critiques on mental practice methodology

Callow, N. and Roberts, R. (2010), 'Imagery: Perspectives, order, and angle', *Psychology of Sport and Exercise*, 4, pp. 325–29.

Roberts, R., Callow, N., Markland, D. and Hardy, L. (2008), 'Assessing imagery ability: The vividness of movement imagery questionnaire – 2', *Journal of Sport and Exercise Psychology*, 30, pp. 200–21.

Callow, N. and Hardy, L. (2005), 'A critical analysis of applied imagery research', in D. Hackfort, J.L. Duda and R. Lidor (eds.), *Handbook of Research in Applied Sport and Exercise Psychology: International Perspectives*, West Virginia: Fitness Information Technology, pp. 21–42.

LeBoutillier, N. and Marks, D.F. (2003), 'Mental imagery and creativity: A meta-analytic review study', *British Journal of Psychology*, 94, 29–44.

McNorgan, C. (2012), "A meta-analytic review of multi-sensory imagery identifies the neural correlates of modality-specific and modality-general imagery", *Frontiers in Human Neuroscience*, 6, pp. 285–302.

References

Ahrabi-Fard, I. (2009), 'Mental practice and attention training: Preparing game player athletes', The American Volleyball Coaches Association Annual Convention, 16 December 2009. http://www.avca.org/includes/media/docs/Mental-Practice-and-Attention-Training-Handout-Page.pdf. Accessed 3 February 2013.

Batson, G. (2004), 'Motor imagery for stroke rehabilitation: Current research as a guide to clinical practice', *Alternative and Complementary Therapies*, 10: 2, pp. 84–89.

Calmels, C., Holmes, P., Lopez, E. and Naman, V. (2006), 'Chronometric comparison of actual and imaged complex movement patterns', *Journal of Motor Behavior*, 38, pp. 339–48.

Carpenter, W.B. (1852), 'On the influence of suggestion in modifying and directing muscular movement, independently of volition', *Proceedings of the Royal Institution of Great Britain*, 12 March 1852, pp. 147–53.

Clark, S., Tremblay, F. and Ste.-Marie, D. (2003), 'Differential modulation of corticospinal excitability during observation, mental imagery and imitation of hand actions', *Neuropsychologia*, 42, pp. 105–12.

Coker Giron, E., McIsaac, T. and Nilsen, D. (2012), 'Effects of kinesthetic versus visual imagery practice on two technical dance movements', *Journal of Dance Medicine and Science*, 16: 1, pp. 36–43.

Decety, J., Jeannerod, M. and Prablanc, C. (1989), 'The timing of mentally represented actions', *Behavioural Brain Research*, 34, pp. 35–42.

Decety, J. (1996a), 'Do imagined and executed actions share the same neural substrate?', *Cognitive Brain Research*, 3, pp. 87–93.

Decety, J. (1996b), 'The neurophysiological basis of motor imagery', *Behavioural Brain Research*, 77, pp. 45–52.

deLahunta, S. and Barnard, B. (2005), 'What's in a Phrase?' in J. Birringer and J. Fenger (eds.), *Tanz im Kopf/Dance and Cognition*, Jahrbuch der Gesellschaft für Tanzforschung 15, Münster: LIT Verlag, pp. 1–14. http://www.choreocog.net/texts/augchoreofindft2_img.pdf. Accessed 3 February 2013.

deLange, F.P., Helmich, R.C. and Toni, I. (2006), 'Posture influences motor imagery: An fMRI study', *NeuroImage*, 33, pp. 609–17.

Deprati, E., Nico, D., Duval, S. and Lacquaniti, F. (2010), 'Different motor imagery modes following brain damage', *Cortex*, 46, pp. 1016–30.

Depraz, N., Varela, F.J., and Vermersch, P. (2003), *On Becoming Aware: A Pragmatics of Experiencing*, Amsterdam, NL: John Benjamins Publishing.

Dickstein, R. and Deutsch, J.E. (2007), 'Motor imagery in physical therapist practice', *Physical Therapy Journal*, 87: 7, pp. 942–53.

Dowd, I. (1995), *Taking Root to Fly: Articles on Functional Anatomy*. Self-published.

Driskell, J.E., Cooper, C. and Moran, A. (1994), 'Does mental practice enhance performance?', *Journal of Applied Psychology*, 79: 4, pp. 481–92.

Feltz, D. and Landers, D. (1983), 'The effects of mental practice on motor skill learning and performance: A meta-analysis', *Journal of Sport Psychology*, 5, pp. 25–57.

Feltz, D.L., Landers, D.M. and Becker, B.J. (1988), 'A revised analysis of the mental practice literature on motor skill learning', *Journal of Experimental Psychology*, 116, pp. 172–91.

Franklin, E. (1996), *Dance Imagery for Technique and Performance,* Champaign, IL: Human Kinetics.

Franklin, E. (2012), *Dynamic Alignment Through Imagery* (2nd edn), Champaign, IL: Human Kinetics.

Gallese, V. (2009), 'Mirror neurons, embodied simulation, and the neural basis of social identification', *Psychoanalytic Dialogues*, 19, pp. 519–36.

Georgopoulos, A.P. and Massey, J.T. (1987), 'Cognitive spatial-motor processes', *Experimental Brain Research*, 65, pp. 361–70.

Goldschmidt, H. (2002), 'Dancing with your head on: Mental imagery techniques for dancers', *Journal of Dance Education*, 2: 1, pp. 15–22.

Granit, R. (1980), *The Purposive Brain*. Cambridge, MA: MIT Classics.

Guillot, A. and Collet, C. (2005), 'Duration of mentally simulated movement: A review', *Journal of Motor Behavior*, 37, pp. 10–20.

Guillot, A. and Collet, C. (2008), 'Construction of the motor imagery integrative model in sport: A review and theoretical investigations of motor imagery use', *International Review of Sport and Exercise Psychology*, 1: 1, pp. 31–44.

Holmes, P. and Calmels, C. (2008), 'A neuroscientific review of imagery and observation use in sport', *Journal of Motor Behavior*, 40: 5, pp. 433–45.

Hugdahl, (2009), 'Overlapping areas of neuronal activation after motor and mental imagery training', *Frontiers in Neuroscience*, 3: 1. http://www.frontiersin.org/Neuroscience/10.3389/neuro.01.008.2009/full. Accessed 13 February 2013.

Jackson, P.L., Lafleur, M.F., Malouin, F., Richards, C. and Doyon, J. (2001), 'Potential role of mental practice using motor imagery in neurologic rehabilitation', *Archives of Physical Medicine and Rehabilitation*, 82: 8, pp. 1133–41.

Jeannerod, M. (1997), *The Cognitive Neuroscience of Action*, Oxford, UK: Blackwell.

Jeannerod, M. (2006), *Motor Cognition: What Actions Tell the Self*, New York, NY: Oxford University Press.

Johnson, S.H. (1998), 'Cerebral organization of motor imagery: Contralateral control of grip selection in mentally representated prehension', *Psychological Science*, 9, pp. 219–22.

Johnson, S.H. (2000), 'Thinking ahead: The case for motor imagery in prospective judgments of prehension', *Cognition*, 74, pp. 33–70.

Jola, C., Angharad, D., and Haggard, P. (2011), 'Proprioceptive integration and body representation: Insights into dancers' expertise', *Experimental Brain Research*, 213: 2–3, pp. 257–65.

Kosslyn, S.M., Thompson, W.L. and Ganis, G. (2006), *The Case for Mental Imagery*, New York, NY: Oxford University Press.

Krasnow, D. and Deveau, J. (2010), *Conditioning With Imagery for Dancers*, Toronto, Ontario, CA: Thompson Educational Publishing.

Lehar, S. (n.d.), 'The representationalism website', http://cns-alumni.bu.edu/~slehar/Representationalism.html. Accessed 13 February 2013.

Lutz, A., Slagter, H.A., Dunne, J.D. and Davidson, R.J. (2008), 'Attention regulation and monitoring in meditation', *Trends in the Cognitive Sciences*, 12: 4, pp. 163–69.

MacIntyre, T. and Moran, A. (2010), 'Meta-imagery processes among elite sports performers' in A. Guillot and C. Collet (eds.), *The Neurophysiological Foundations of Mental and Motor Imagery*, Oxford, UK: Oxford University Press, pp. 227–44.

McCullagh, P. and Weiss, M.R. (2001), 'Modeling: Considerations for motor skill performance and psychological responses' in R.N. Singer, H.A. Hausenblaus and C.M. Janelle (eds.), *Handbook of Sport Psychology* (2nd edn), New York, NY: Wiley, pp. 205–38.

Magali, L., Guillot, A., Maton, S., Doyon, J. and Collet, C. (2008), 'Effect of imagined movement speed on subsequent motor performance', *Journal of Motor Behavior*, 40: 2, pp. 117–32.

May, J., Calvo-Merino, B., deLahunta, S. et al. (2011), 'Points in mental space: An interdisciplinary study of imagery in movement creation', *Dance Research Journal*, 29: 2, pp. 404–32.

McNorgan, C. (2012), 'A meta-analytic review of multi-sensory identifies the neural correlates of modality-specific and modality-general imagery', *Frontiers in Human Neuroscience*, 6, pp. 285–302.

Moran, A. (2009), 'Cognitive psychology in sport: Progress and prospects', *Psychology of Sport and Exercise*, 10, pp. 420–26.

Moran, A., Guillot, A., MacIntyre, T. and Collet, C. (2012), 'Re-imagining motor imagery: Building bridges between cognitive neuroscience and sport psychology', *British Journal of Psychology*, 103, pp. 224–47.

Morris, T., Spittle, M. and Watt, A.P. (2005), *Imagery in Sport*, Leeds, UK: Human Kinetics.

Moulton, S.T. and Kosslyn, S.M. (2009), 'Imagining predictions: Mental imagery as mental emulation', *Philosophical Transactions of the Royal Society, B: Biological Sciences*, 364, pp. 1273–80.

Mulder, T. (2007), 'Motor imagery and action observation: Cognitive tools for rehabilitation', *Journal of Neural Transmission*, 114: 10, pp. 1265–78.

Murphy, S. and Martin, K. (2002), 'The use of imagery in sport' in T. Horn (ed.), *Advances in Sport Psychology* (2nd edn), Champaign, IL: Human Kinetics, pp. 405–39.

Murphy, S.M., Nordin, S. and Cumming, J. (2008), 'Imagery in sport, exercise, and dance' in T.S. Horn (ed.), *Advances in Sport Psychology* (3rd edn), Champaign, IL: Human Kinetics, pp. 297–324.

Nordin, S.M. and Cumming, J. (2007), 'Where, when, and how: A quantitative account of dance imagery', *Research Quarterly for Exercise in Sport*, 78: 4, pp. 390–95.

Nordin, S.M. and Cumming, J. (2005), 'Professional dancers describe their imagery: Where, when, what, why and how', *The Sport Psychologist*, 19, pp. 395–416.

Pearson, D.G., Deeprose, C., Wallace-Hadrill, S.M.A., Burnett Heyes, S. and Holmes, E.A. (2013), 'Assessing mental imagery in clinical psychology: A review of imagery measures and a guiding framework', *Clinical Psychology Review*, 33: 1, pp. 1–23.

Rosenbaum, D.A. Meulenbroek, R.G.J. and Vaughan, J. (2004), 'What is the point of motor planning', *International Journal of Sport and Exercise Psychology*, 2, pp. 439–69.

Samuels, M. and Samuels, N. (1975), *Seeing With the Mind's Eye: The History, Techniques and Uses of Visualization*, New York, NY: Random House.

Sheets-Johnstone, M. (2009), *The Corporeal Turn: An Interdisciplinary Reader*, Exeter, UK: Imprint Academic.

Sheets-Johnstone, M. (2010), 'Thinking in movement: Further analyses and validations', in J. Stewart, O. Gapenne and E.A. Di Paolo (eds.), *Enaction: Toward New Paradigm for Cognitive Science*, Cambridge, MA: MIT Press, pp. 165–181.

Sweigard, L. (1974), *Human Movement Potential: Its Ideokinetic Facilitation*, New York, NY: Dodd Mead.

Thinus-Blanc, C. and Gaunet, F. (1999), 'Spatial processing in animals and humans: The organizing function of representations for information gathering', in R.G. Golledge (ed.), *Wayfinding Behavior: Cognitive Mapping and Other Spatial Processes*, Baltimore, MD: The Johns Hopkins Press, pp. 294–307.

Travis, F. and Shear, J. (2010), 'Focused attention, open monitoring and automatic self-transcending: Categories to organize meditations from Vedic, Buddhist and Chinese traditions', *Conscious Cognition*, 19: 4, pp. 1110–18.

Notes

1   Looking primarily at neural processes, the mind either can *represent* or *simulate* experience (Moran et al. 2012). A representation is something that *stands in* for experience, like a mental construct (either concrete or abstract) (Lehar n.d.). Simulation, on the other hand,

suggests covertly performing what we observe, thereby acting as if we are also doing the same thing we observe (Gallese 2009). Simulation usually implies empathy. Both formulations arguably carry 'kinematic content' and, therefore, are 'motor' acts (Jeannerod 2006: 24). The debate over whether the brain 'represents' or 'simulates' movement (action) is unresolved. See Lehar, S. (nd), 'The representationalism web site' http://cns-alumni.bu.edu/~slehar/Representationalism.html, and Frasca, G. (2001), 'Simulation 101: Simulation versus representation, http://www.ludology.org/articles/sim1/simulation101.html.

2   See the website on Ideokinesis at http://www.ideokinesis.com/. Meta-analyses from sports and neuroscience are listed in the references.

3   For the purposes of this discussion, we'll use the term MPMI to include mentally visualizing anatomical structures (typical to Ideokinesis), although differences exist between both techniques. For a discussion of the differences from a dance perspective, see http://www.indefocus.com/articles/featured-articles/222-the-use-of-imagery-and-visualisation-in-contemporary-dance.

4   Within neuroscience, the 'agent' is considered either a *representation* (or mental construct) in the brain or a *simulation* of actual experience (Moran et al. 2012). See endnote 1 and subsequent quotes from Sheets-Johnstone.

5   From the perspective of Sweigard Ideokinesis, the effectiveness in motor-skill training comes from practicing the images in the constructive rest position (Sweigard 1974). This meant practicing a skill covertly, visually perceiving motor imagery explicitly and clearly. Mentally, the motor images should *move*. Sweigard and Clark suggested 20 minutes of imagery practice to re-educate posture and coordination. This time period issued out of their empirical research. Sports coaches also provide guidelines for training attention through mental practice (Ahrabi-Fard 2009), although the intention is aimed more at psychological coping than neuromuscular re-education.

Chapter 9

Somatic Approaches to Training Attention: Part II
Somatic Grounding

Poise is a balanced concentration immediately prior to action. It is the a priori of a self-aware act. Poise itself is an action, but one of a wholly different kind. It differs from ordinary undertakings in point of origination, intention, quality of attention, rhythm, and reason. Poise is the response of awareness to the call of a situation...Before poise can reveal itself, a tension that is the psychophysical milieu of accomplishment must ease...All evidence suggests that poise is not the natural outgrowth of a process that begins in distraction, preoccupation, and insensitivity.

(Applebaum 1992: 78)

Overview – Somatic Grounding (SG)

The last three chapters have addressed embodied attention and its relationship to enhancing physical performance. Chapter 6 introduced the topic of the inter-relationship between attention and effort in skilled performance. Chapter 7 described commonalities in the somatic learning milieu that are conducive to training embodied attention. Chapter 8 provided an update on the mental practice of motor imagery (MPMI) and challenges facing research and training of visual attention.

This chapter introduces another somatic pathway into attention training: *Somatic Grounding* (SG). We invented the term 'Somatic Grounding' to describe a process of attending to sensations arising from bodily surface contact and movement within gravity. In MPMI, persons focus attention on mentally envisioning moving images, in SG, persons attend to sensations arising from touch and movement (i.e., tactile-kinesthetic sensations and related images). In this respect, MPMI primarily is a *feed-forward* model of motor learning. SG is a *feedback* model.

Below, we describe a particular SG exercise designed to sensitize the dancer/mover's awareness to postural reactions underlying verticality and balance. The exercise is an experience in controlled falling and recovering. The dancer/mover lies prone on a novel surface and slowly performs a series of small-range trunk movements toward and away from gravity. The exercise affords two major benefits: first, dancers can focus sensitively on input from 'graviceptors' (Mittlestaedt 1996: 55) – sensations arising from skin, muscles, fascia, organs and other bodily tissues from moving in gravity. Developmentally (that is, throughout life) these tactile-kinesthetic sensations inform us about tension, pressure, texture, velocity and other embodied knowledge essential to maintaining poised verticality and balance. By practicing the exercise, the dancer/mover can gain an embodied sense of the importance of the midline of the trunk and the anterior body wall in upright balance.

Second, the exercise is designed to re-educate neuromuscular patterns to improve trunk stability and balance. It is performed slowly and attentively enough to notice postural reactions in response to small disturbances of balance. When the body starts to fall (even when that incipient fall is self-initiated), global reflex patterns (muscular synergies) arise throughout the body. The controlled learning environment in SG offers an inroad to identifying and re-educating maladaptive reflex reactions to balance disturbances. By practicing and reflecting on the exercise, dancers can learn more flexible embodied responses.

Neuroscientific evidence is limited supporting the utility of somatic methods for retraining postural control and balance. While limited behavioral data exists on the effectiveness of MPMI for postural retraining,[1] studies utilizing somatosensory approaches to improving balance are nearly non-existent. This omission derives partly from the difficulty in isolating somatosensory input from visual- and other sensory data.

Rather than quantitative evidence, however, we base this exercise design primarily on empirical evidence from various somatic practices as well as from theories on motor developmental theory and dynamical systems. Based on our teaching experience, we speculate that SG offers the mover conscious access to his or her habitual (stereotypic) balance responses. Improvements may carry over to postural support in standing, but more research is needed in this area. We suggest first trying the exercise in four stages:

1. Perform the pre-test (the 'Experiential prelude' below) (~5–10 minutes).
2. Complete the SG exercise with several variations (~30 minutes).
3. Repeat the pre-test for a post-test comparison (~5 minutes).
4. Reflect on the experience, both in the moment and throughout the day.

Experiential prelude

The following exercise is a *pre-test*. A pre-test is a useful way to compare the before-and-after effects of an exercise. It will help establish a baseline of how well you do before and after completing the *SG exercise* described in this chapter. The exercise is a step from classical ballet vocabulary – the battement tendu.[2] Here, we choose the tendu as a test of dynamic balance. We've also adapted the exercise for non-dancers. Complete the pre-test exercise before practicing the SG exercise.

Dancers: find an unobstructed space about 10' × 10'. Stand in ballet first position on a wooden floor (no carpet), with your arms in second position. Perform four battement tendus en avante with the right foot (Photo 9.1). Execute the four tendus slowly, taking approximately 10 seconds per limb to complete the movement. Immediately, repeat the sequence with your left foot. Notice how you do this – how you come to standing, how

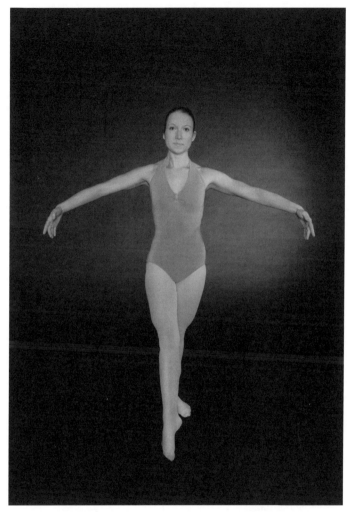

Photo 9.1: Tendu en avant (photo credit. Ludwig Photography).

you distribute your weight over each foot, how you initiate the movement, how your trunk shifts in advancing each leg, the sensations connected with arm and trunk support, your gaze and any other pertinent observations. Record the details of your experience on a piece of paper. Rate your pre-test experience in terms of proficiency and ease of accomplishment and balance. Use the criteria on the rating sheet, if you would prefer (Chart 9.1). A rating of 1 suggests *poorly executed* performance and a rating of 5 indicates your *best* performance. After completing the SG exercise, repeat the pre-test series of tendus. Rate yourself again. Compare your pre-test impressions with your immediate 'post-test' impressions.

Chart 9.1: Experiential prelude rating scale for the battement tendu

Scoring (scale of 1 to 5): 1 = worst performance, 5 = best

Movement Phases	Pre-test	Post-test	Comments
Assumption of position			
Initiating the tendu			
Reaching the toe to the end point			
Reversing and restoring original position			
Changing sides			

Suggested criteria

1 = poorly executed

- Hesitancy in assuming the position
- Excessive shifting of weight from foot to foot to stabilize in stance
- Postural malalignment
- Backward tilt of the torso as leg advances
- Torso wobbling as leg moves in either direction (forward or backward)
- Excessive lateral shift of the torso in changing feet
- Arm fatigue at any point in the exercise
- Holding the breath
- Focus and head rigidly fixed

5 = best performance

- Feeling of ease and support in assuming the position
- Noticeable freedom of breathing
- Entire torso quiet and stable without wobbling throughout
- No signs of fatigue
- Focus free to move
- Feeling of freedom to move any body part in any direction on command

Non-dancers: Conduct the same experiment. Stand in your stocking feet on a non-carpeted floor with your heels together and your toes slightly turned out, knees extended. Support your arms out to your sides at shoulder level. Stand firmly on your left leg and advance the right foot (toes) along the floor as far as it will go. Then, bring it back. Repeat with the other foot. Keep to the same tempo (~10 seconds per leg). Use a stopwatch or metronome, if you need to keep an external timekeeper. Record your experience as best as you can – the sensations, feelings and ease of balancing to accomplish these leg movements. Use the rating chart for guidelines. After practicing the SG exercise described in the chapter, repeat the pre-test. Compare your before-and-after experience.

SG – scientific rationale

Throughout all stages of growth and development, we learn to move in gravity, exploring the flow of our weight as our body shapes and navigates in and out of a vertical world. Our first 'consciousness' is 'corporeal' (Sheets-Johnstone 2011: 62–63). Our 'sensate-tactile-kinesthetic body' is fundamental to meeting gravity and learning to stand upright. Moreover, humans embody 'sentience',…'the feeling of being alive and exercising effort in movement' (Thompson 2007: 229, 231). The 'sensate-tactile-kinesthetic body' is 'a body rich in movement memories, expectations, and values, a body that has in consequence developed certain kinetic dispositions, habits, and ways of responding' (Sheets-Johnstone 2011: 382).[3] We make sense of the world by coming into direct contact with it – by touching and being touched back (Reed 1996). This profound sensitivity to this tactile information is the baseline for building a capacity for human attunement, attachment and bonding, and the precursor of empathy and embodied consciousness (Berrol 2006; Bainbridge-Cohen 2012).

To underscore the potential effectiveness of the SG exercise, however, we'll focus mainly on balance. Balance emerges from integrated sensory acuity and the timely and appropriate responses of the neuromuscular system to balance disturbances.[4] Dynamic control of upright posture first requires sensory sensibility in meeting gravity. The integrated input from visual, vestibular and somatosensory systems provides a powerful reference for upright orientation and balance (Karnath, Ferber and Dichgans 2000; Massion, Alexandrov and Frolov 2004; Horak 2006; Morningstar et al. 2005). In this discussion on balance, we focus on somatosensory 'graviception' (Mittlestaedt 1996). 'Graviceptors' are sensory receptors – tactile and proprioceptive mechanoreceptors and baroreceptors (pressure receptors) (ibid.: 55). Graviceptors are extremely abundant (redundant) throughout the body's surface and interior. Graviceptors are somatosensory afferent nerves from cutaneous (skin) and fascial receptors, muscle spindles and golgi tendon organs, joint afferents. A 'proprioceptive chain' of somatosensory receptors runs from head to toe, including the extraocular muscles in the eyes, neck, trunk, hands, legs and feet (Roll and Roll 1988). In addition, autonomic organs regulation (heart and blood vessels, for example) help regulate balance. These sensory organs generate neural signals that encode for the vector of gravity (Binder, Hirokawa and Windhorst 2009) ensuring a sound body-to-earth relationship.

Our perception of gravitational vertical, for example, is remarkably accurate under normal circumstances, that is, free from adventitious circumstances, such as disease (stroke) or environmental challenges (surfing) or anomalies (trick mirrors). Normally, the sense of upright vertical is so accurate that we can readily detect tilting when our body is less than two-degrees off-center. Our sense of the *vertical* varies, though, depending on where we are in space. Orientation is flexible and learned, formed by sensory encoding to different environments. These codes are integrated in the nervous system to provide a unified spatial picture of right relationship to the environment. With practice, we can adjust physiologically to any orientation – standing right side up, sideways or upside down.

Graviception helps explain the essential role of the trunk in balance. Trunk maturation leads human motor development and control from birth through adolescence. Gradual support for the head and spine in gravity precedes that of the limbs in all aspects of functional support – reaching, walking etc. (Assaiante and Amblard 1995). Control is not only a function of reflex synergy patterns,[5] but also the sensorimotor coordination of the superficial and deep muscles. These muscles have unique properties of responsiveness integral to bodily support and balance (Moseley, Hodges and Gandevia 2002). The most proximal muscles (e.g., deep spinal muscles) assume the main task of postural support. Larger, more superficial muscles remain comparatively free to engage in large range, voluntary trunk movements (Sweigard 1974). These deeper muscles are usually smaller and not under conscious control. They are richly innervated with sensory nerves for proprioception. These muscles are considered *involuntary* (that is, less accessible by conscious will) (Long and Fortin 2012).

A number of somatic approaches train balance by emphasizing improved muscular balance between superficial and deep muscles of the trunk, such as the Feldenkrais Method, the Alexander Technique and Body-Mind Centering (Long and Fortin 2012; Cacciatore et al. 2010; Bainbridge-Cohen 2012). This process of accessing deeper muscles is not a matter of strengthening them. Rather, the process involves becoming consciously aware of sensations arising from body-to-surface-contact within situations of fall risk. Human systems develop at different rates and in different areas of the same body part (Thelen 1995; Thelen and Smith 1994). The trunk generally stabilizes and matures before the limbs. This implies more proximal control (trunk stability) before distal control (using hands and feet). Trunk control provides a stable frame of reference for orientation and facing, midline organization, body segment divisions and for cognitive development as well as functional and social viability (Assaiante et al. 2005). If the trunk is stable against the movement of the arms and legs, an infant can master skills more readily – incidental movements, goal-directed actions and social interactions. Developmentally, the movement of the lower pelvis precedes that of the shoulders and the shoulders precedes the head for a stable succession toward upright walking (Hodges et al. 2000). Up to age ten, for example, arm movement is usually coupled tightly with trunk movement, often unable to move in differentiated patterns (Ting and McKay 2007). Dance teachers observe this phenomenon, for example, when children's arms mimic their leg movement during pliés, flexing and extending at the same time.

The SG exercise described below is designed to stimulate the anterior surface of the trunk and midline by lying on the belly (prone). This exercise affords the dancer/mover an experience of falling safely. Balance responses often go unnoticed, masked by the pace and size of everyday movement and our usual focus on the task (rather than the body's sensations). Here, the exercise can be performed done slowly and sensitively enough to disturb the learner's sense of equilibrium and safety. In SG, dancer/movers are asked to focus their attention on discrete sensations in response to voluntarily shifting portions of the trunk off the bolster. With these constraints, dancer/movers can learn to distinguish more subtle messages coming from disturbances of balance. The balance disturbance in this context is a small-range voluntary movement, slowly performed on a large bolster. (Preparation, 9.2).

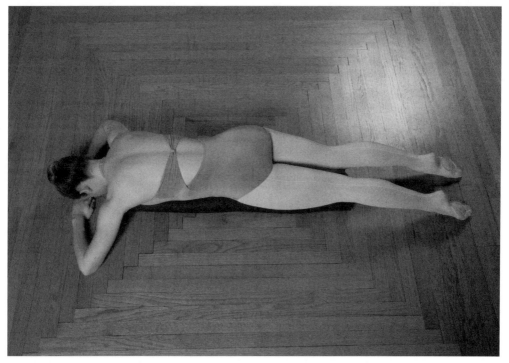

Photo 9.2: Preparation: Prone on bolster (photo credit. Ludwig Photography).

The mover initiates an incrementally small lateral shift of the pelvis (a voluntary self-perturbation, 9.3). The shift first is in the direction of gravity (towards the floor) and then away from gravity (remounting the bolster). The mover sensitively attends to these phases toward and away from gravity. Tactile-kinesthetic sensations arise from bodily movement in gravity. Additionally, the exercise can induce tension in the trunk from changes in pressure, speed, inertia, friction and a variety of other gravitational effects. The *small fall* activates global synergy patterns within the trunk and limbs. By keeping the focus of attention

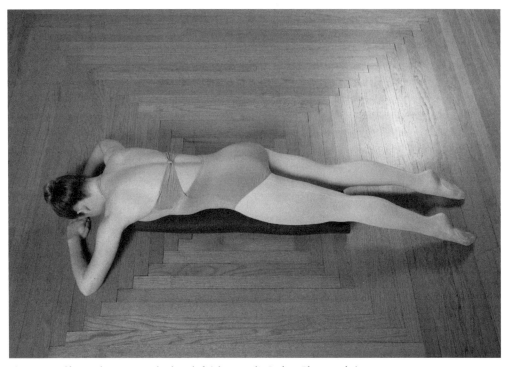

Photo 9.3: Self-Perturbation: Lateral pelvic shift (photo credit. Ludwig Photography).

lively throughout the exercise, movers can detect sensations not readily perceived in larger movement experiences.

The suggested time frame for completing the exercise is approximately 30–40 minutes. There is an old Zen adage that says you should sit for twenty minutes a day unless you are too busy; then you should sit for an hour (unknown). It appears that twenty minutes is a minimum of time needed to engage self-regulatory processes. These processes quiet mental distractions and intensify the focus on states of embodiment. Such explorations gradually expand the 'perceptual-motor workspace' or movement envelope, facilitating a change in consciousness (Newell, McDonald and Kugler 1991; Buchanan and Ulrich 2001).[6]

An example of a more challenging experience than the SG exercise exists in the Contact Improvisation lexicon: Steve Paxton's 'Small Dance' (1986/2009). Paxton's self-guided exploration of standing opens attention to the many small oscillations of the limbs to maintain the body upright. I have adapted Paxton's small dance for students in various classes I've taught in Somatics. Many find this exploration challenging, particularly if they have not been exposed to somatic trainings where sensory awareness is augmented and effort is reduced (Batson 2010).

Paxton (1986/2009) offers a number of insights into how standing is a small dance:

- 'The small dance is a continuous exploration of the least muscular effort necessary to maintain a moveable vertical alignment;
- the small dance is listening to how the body reflexes communicate with gravity, muscles, and bones to stay in an effortless continuously changing alignment;
- the small dance is listening to how gravity invites the bones to find the best possible alignment in each moment;
- the small dance is standing. Standing is inviting gravity to align the bones'.

The exercise in SG is performed with the trunk supported on a large bolster approximately 8–12 inches (20.3–30.5 cm) in thickness (Photo 9.2 and Photo 9.3). You can make this bolster easily by rolling up a large, stiff blanket. The rationale for this particular setup includes:

- Prone as opposed to supine (a gravity-assisted position that helps induce physiological flexion by anterior surface contact with the floor/ground) (Bainbridge-Cohen 2012).
- Prone positioning stabilizes the trunk and other body segments in a gravity-minimized environment.
- Contact of the front surface of the body with a compliant surface that is elevated approximately one foot off the ground. The spine is in a horizontal relationship to gravity. Here, the anterior surfaces of the organs hang toward gravity. This enhances the tactile stimulation to the anterior trunk along with facilitating the emergence of other more subtle responses to perturbations.
- The face/eyes are relieved of orienting and perceiving.
- The trunk acts as primary mover of the body before the limbs.
- Upper and lower limbs are freed from doing tasks and help support the trunk.
- The developmental sequence can be replicated through movement exploration – midline, body half, ipsi/contralateral, homologous and homolateral movements.
- Controlled falling (toward gravity) and restoring stability of the trunk (away from gravity) is safe and low to the ground. At the same time, the position still is high enough off the ground to perturb balance.
- The process of exploration becomes more important than the movements performed.

Guidelines

Do not use a foam roller for this exercise. The surface is too hard and the roller too mobile! Wear comfortable, soft clothing that can slide easily on the bolster.

Lie prone on the bolster (on your stomach), and put your forehead on your hands so that your head is in midline (Photo 9.2). This bolster should support your midline in prone from your sternum to a few inches beyond your pubic bone. Your head should be off the end of the bolster. Position your legs so that the weight is on the dorsum of both feet (more or less in parallel) without a lot of external or internal rotation at the hip joints, if possible. Once situated on the bolster, the mover needs to take several minutes tuning into bodily sensations in stillness. Take five full minutes to notice the buzz inside your head as you just let your thinking settle down to focus quietly on arising sensations. Resist naming them at first. What's making contact with the bolster? What's contacting the floor? Can you let go of unnecessary effort and allow the surface contact to support?

Once you have quieted your thinking, notice how breathing is shaping the torso and its contact with the bolster – the location of breath, its rate, rhythm and depth, and its in and out phases. Notice the directional pulls in your body in relation to breathing and to the contact with the floor. Where are the pressures in the contact and how do they change with the breathing cycle? Does your inhale take the chest closer to the soft cylinder of the blanket, or further away, for example?

First practice the exercise mentally only. Inhibit the intention to actually move. *Think* you are going to shift your pelvis off the bolster to the right no more than 1–2 inches. Pause in your thinking, and then *restore* your pelvis in your mind to the midline. Repeat the visualization to the left. Notice the differences, simply with thinking. What are you doing with your gaze? Are you *watching* your pelvis move? Can you simply *sense* your pelvis moving without searching for it?

Pause and rest for a minute or so. When you begin to actually move, move very slowly, gently and with attention to the tactile and other movement dynamics of the journey. Go slowly enough to observe the details and try for yourself to identify as many different phases as you can that go into executing the step, from assumption of first position to the termination of the whole movement series.

Slide your pelvis to the right no more than 1–2 inches (3–5 cm) in the direction of gravity – no more (9.3)! Pay attention to the duration between the thought of moving and actually initiating the movement. Pay attention to how you slide your pelvis. Avoid speed and abrupt movements. Pause at the end of the movement and suspend as gravity pulls on your lower trunk. Choose when you wish to restore your pelvis back to where it started. Notice the effort it takes to restore the starting position.

Repeat this movement several times. After about 5 minutes of ex-centering and restoring your pelvis toward the right, rest on the bolster. You can roll off of it, if you are uncomfortable, but really rest for 3 to 4 minutes until you feel ready enough to reflect on this phase of the exercise.

Before repeating the exercise to the left, consider the following questions (or perhaps just record your own inquiry):

1. What sensations arise with the thought of moving?
2. How do these sensations change as you actually start to move?
3. How readily can you identify what initiates the movement?
4. How easy is it for you to move in the direction of gravity? What happens in the different aspects of the trunk (front, back, sides), when you shifted?
5. How easy was it for you to restore your position?

6. How far do you travel readily and comfortably?
7. In what direction does your upper trunk shift as you move your pelvis? Does it go down and forward, up and back, or rotate slightly?
8. What do you feel in your neck and upper back when you come into position and raise the arms? A pulling down in the chest? An arching of the lumbar spine?
9. What happens to your breathing as you start to move? At other points in the sequence?
10. What happens when you shift the pelvis to the opposite side? How does the body stabilize? Does this difference between sides coincide with technical issues you have in dance class?
11. Describe the quality of the weight shift in the direction of gravity – e.g., abrupt and halting, or smooth and sustained.
12. What happens in your body at the moment of reversing the movement?
13. What muscles release as you let go of the movement and rest?
14. Describe the state of your embodiment after practicing the one side.

You can repeat the exercise, adding any of the following variations to the basic structure:

1. Do the same exercise shifting your upper torso. Compare the differences.
2. Try shifting the upper and lower trunk as one unit (log roll); or, try counterbalancing the upper and lower trunk segments, one going one direction, one the other.
3. Move your eyes with your pelvis/thorax. The point is to feel the *movement* of the eyes, neither trying to see anything, nor increasing your range of eye motion. Moving the eyes in non-habitual patterns may illuminate how easily our eyes habituate to various patterns in helping stabilize balance.
4. Vary your attention to different tissues – what difference does it make to focus on bones, for example. Here, the exercise is a lesson in leverage. Or, perhaps choose another body-mind centering system exploration – lungs, fluids, glands etc. (Bainbridge-Cohen 2012).
5. Identify a maladaptive postural habit you wish to re-educate and practice the same exercise daily for a month. See what the results are with continued practice.

Once you have spent at least 30 minutes exploring this exercise, stand and repeat that first pre-test. What differences do you sense?

If you are a dancer, you can play with executing the tendu in a host of other novel contexts. For example, you can try various body contact explorations, such as trying the tendu in sidelying or partnering with someone back-to-back. Another challenge might be to perform the tendu upside-down. For safety, start the practice in the familiar yoga position of downward-facing dog. Try a few tendus from this position. In being upside-down, you can experience ground reaction force coming through the arms and upper body, a great way to strengthen upper-body support. As you move to the wall, make sure you have a partner to spot you as you assume the 90-degree jackknife position with your feet on the wall. Once stabilized on your hands and arms, try your tendu here. Practice advancing your leg (i.e., controlling the fall of your leg) no more than a few degrees until you feel safe and stable enough to allow a larger arc of movement. You should be able to breathe, talk and sing with ease. Once you've tried a couple tendu variations, check in with your baseline standing tendu again. Rate your performance again. Record your reflections. What has changed/improved? As you enter back in to technique class, see what you can recall from these somatic-based practices that can assist you as your explore various themes and variations (Batson 2010).

Expanding the exercise phases

Another useful reflective exercise it to name all the different movement phases involved in the basic SG exercise. Each phase is an important interval for learning. Learners can amplify attention to embodied experience in each phase. Each phase can offer new insights into embodied knowledge. Some of the phases are listed below. Feel free to add others.

1. Assuming the position (lying face down on the bolster, or sidelying, as another option).
2. Sensory attunement – the shift from busy brain to focused sensory awareness.
3. Body scanning (sensing the base of support…e.g., what's touching the floor).
4. Pre-initiation (having the intention to move, and noticing how the body reacts).
5. The onset of initiation – slow, small-range (the first awareness of effort and refinement of that effort).
6. Weight shift and transfer to facilitate the advancement of the gesturing pelvis or upper torso.
7. Sequencing to the decided end range of the movement.
8. The moment of deciding to reverse the movement and return to the starting position.
9. Sensing the ascent of the pelvis.
10. Sensing the moments of rebalancing in midline.
11. Letting the weight descend into rest (slowly restoring the preparatory position).
12. Fully resting (the point at which no sensations of movement execution linger).

Summary

Somatic approaches can help dancers understand the importance of trunk integration for stabilization and balance. Postural control problems can become obscured by skilled compensation and strength during real time execution. The SG exercise trains embodied attention by attuning to the more hidden tactile and kinesthetic dynamics underlying balance. The authors have researched this exploration in a variety of empirical contexts, but not as formal research. The full effects of this exercise and their carryover into technique await further investigation.

References

Applebaum, D. (1992), *The Stop*, New York, NY: Peter Lang.

Assaiante, C. and Amblard, B. (1995), 'An ontogenetic model for the sensorimotor organization of balance control in humans', *Human Movement Science*, 14, pp. 13–43.

Assaiante, C., Mallau, S., Sebastien, V., Jover, M. and Schmitz, C. (2005), 'Development of postural control in healthy children: A functional approach', *Neural Plasticity*, 12, pp. 109–18.

Bainbridge-Cohen, B. (2012), *Sensing, Feeling and Action: The Experiential Anatomy of Body-Mind Centering*, 3rd edn, Northampton, MA: Contact Editions.

Batson, G. (2010), 'Understanding balance: Applying science to dance training', *The IADMS Bulletin for Teachers*, 2: 1, pp. 14–16. http://www.iadms.org. Accessed 14 February 2013.

Bernstein, N. (1967), *The Co-ordination and Regulation of Movements*, Oxford, UK: Pergamon Press.

Berrol, C.F. (2006), 'Neuroscience meets dance/movement therapy: Mirror neurons, the therapeutic process and empathy', *The Arts in Psychotherapy*, 33: 4, pp. 302–15.

Binder, M.D., Hirokawa, N. and Windhorst, U. (eds.) (2009), *Encyclopedia of Neuroscience*, Vol. 2, New York, NY: Springer.

Buchanan, P.A. and Ulrich, B.D. (2001), 'The Feldenkrais Method: A dynamic approach to changing motor behavior', *Research Quarterly for Exercise and Sport*, 72: 4, pp. 315–23.

Cacciatore, T.W., Gurfinkel, V.S., Horak, F.B., Cordo, P.J. and Ames, K.E. (2010), 'Increased dynamic regulation of postural tone through Alexander Technique training', *Human Movement Science*, 30: 1, pp. 74–89.

Fairweather, M.M. and Sidaway, B. (1993), 'Ideokinetic imagery as a postural development technique', *Research Quarterly for Exercise and Sport*, 64: 4, pp. 385–92.

Hodges, P.W., Cresswell, A.G., Daggfeldt, K. and Thorstensson, A. (2000), 'Three dimensional preparatory trunk motion precedes asymmetrical upper limb movement', *Gait and Posture*, 11: 2, pp. 92–101.

Horak, F.B. (2006), 'Postural orientation and equilibrium: What do we need to know about neural control of balance to prevent falls?', *Age Ageing*, 35: 2, pp. ii7–ii11.

Huelster, L. (1949), *The Relationship Between Bilateral Contour Asymmetry in the Human Body in Standing and Walking*, Unpublished Ph.D. Thesis, New York University, School of Education.

Huelster, L. (1953), 'The relationship between bilateral contour asymmetry in the human body in standing and walking', *Research Quarterly American Association of Health and Physical Education*, 24, pp. 44–55.

Karnath, H.O., Ferber, S. and Dichgans, J. (2000), 'The origins of contraversive pushing: Evidence for a second graviceptive system in humans', *Neurology*, 55, pp. 1298–304.

Long, W. and Fortin, S. (2012), *Integrating the Feldenkrais Method within the dance classroom*. http://ebookbrowse.com/warwick-long-sylvie-fortin-dance-pdf-d361919073. Accessed 20 January 2013.

Massion, J., Alexandrov, A. and Frolov, A. (2004), 'Why and how are posture and movement coordinated?', *Progress in Brain Research*, 143, pp. 13–27.

Mittlestaedt, H. (1996), 'Somatic graviception', *Biological Psychology*, 42, pp. 53–74.

Mittlestaedt, H. (1998), 'Origin and processing of postural information', *Neuroscience Biobehavioral Reviews*, 22, pp. 473–78.

Morningstar, M.W., Pettibon, B.R., Schlappi, H., Schlappi, M. and Ireland, T.V. (2005), 'Reflex control of the spine and posture: A review of the literature from a chiropractic perspective', *Chiropractic and Osteopathy*, 13, pp. 16–22.

Moseley, G.L., Hodges, P.W. and Gandevia, S.C. (2002), 'Deep and superficial fibers of the lumbar multifidus muscle are differentially active during voluntary arm movements', *Spine*, 27: 2, pp. 29–36.

Newell, K.M., McDonald, P.V. and Kugler, P.N. (1991), 'The perceptual-motor workspace and the acquisition of skill', in J. Requin and G.E. Stelmach (eds.), *Tutorials in Motor Neuroscience*, Amsterdam: Kluwer Academic Publishers, pp. 95–108.

Paxton, S. (1986/2009), talk by Steve Paxton at CI36, Contact Improvisation's 36th Birthday Celebration in Huntingdon, PA, 13 June 2008. Reprinted from *Contact Quarterly*, 34: 1, Winter/Spring 2009. http://www.contactquarterly.com/cq/webtext/Paxtontalk.html. Accessed 13 December 2012.

Reed, E.S. (1996), *Encountering the World: Toward an Ecological Psychology*, New York, NY: Oxford University Press.

Roll, J.P. and Roll, R. (1988), 'From eye to foot: A proprioceptive chain involved in postural control' in B. Amblard, A. Berthoz and F. Clarac (eds.), *Posture and Gait: Development, Adaptation and Modulation*, Amsterdam: Elsevier, pp. 155–64.

Sheets-Johnstone, M. (2011), *The Primacy of Movement*, 2nd edn, Philadelphia, PA: John Benjamins Publishing Company.

Sweigard, L. (1974), *Human Movement Potential: Its Ideokinetic Facilitation*. Boston, MA: Addison-Wesley Educational Publishers.

Thelen, E. (1995), 'Motor development: A new synthesis', *American Psychologist*, 50: 2, pp. 79–95.

Thelen, E. and Smith, L.B. (1994), *A Dynamics Systems Approach to the Development of Cognition and Action*, Cambridge, MA: Bradford Books/MIT Press.

Thompson, E. (2007), *Mind in Life: Biology, Phenomenology and the Sciences of Mind*. Cambridge, MA: Harvard University Press.

Ting, L.H. and McKay, J.L. (2007), 'Neuromechanics of muscle synergies for posture and movement', *Current Opinion in Neurobiology*, 17, pp. 622–28.

Notes

1   Few research studies exist from the late twentieth century to date examining the effectiveness of Ideokinesis on postural control. A few studies exist on postural improvement (Huelster 1949; Huelster 1953; Fairweather and Sidaway 1993). These address improvements in biomechanical alignment rather than showing the effectiveness of Ideokinesis in re-educating neuromuscular reflex responses integral to training balance. A fuller bibliography can be found at http://www.ideokinesis.com/bibliography/bibliography.htm. See below for research examples on the effects of the Alexander Technique or the Feldenkrais Method® on balance.

2   The concept for this chapter evolved from an article by Batson (2010): 'Improving postural control in the battement tendu: One teacher's reflections and somatic exercises', *Journal of Dance Education*, 10: 1, pp. 6–13. Batson designed the SG exercise described here as a prelude to enhancing postural control of the trunk to support the battement tendu. Likeness to any other exercise(s) is coincidental. See Appendix 1 for an expanded primer on balance that originally served as the theoretical baseline for this article.

3   Sheets-Johnstone expounds on the importance of tactile-kinesthesthetic consciousness and intercorporeality at great length throughout her book (2011).

4   This chapter will focus on sensory graviceptors. See Appendix 1 for a description of neuromuscular synergy patterns and balance.

5   Trunk maturation is an enormous subject and too complex to go into depth here. Suffice to say that the first sign of maturation in infancy is the development of fast-acting neuromuscular response patterns in the trunk, known as *synergies* (Massion, Alexandrov and Frolov 2004; Bernstein 1967). Balance disturbances demand fast-acting synergistic activation of the trunk in babies. If these patterns are impaired, they may limit the timely developmental transition from sitting to independent walking (Assaiante and Amblard 1995). Poorly coordinated or underdeveloped postural control is seen in excessive agonist-antagonist fixation (co-activation) of the trunk- or other limb muscles. This results in lack of differentiated movement between trunk and limbs and awkward movement transitions. Again, see Appendix 1 for an explanation of synergy patterns.

6   Any similarities of this exercise to a Feldenkrais Awareness Through Movement™ (ATM) lesson are coincidental. If the exercise context appears in the ATM archive, it is unknown to the author. The exploratory process shares similarities in the process of attending, certainly. Learning elements include attending to sensory feedback from self-induced, small-range movement perturbations; curiosity rather than directed toward a specific goal; slow pacing; refraining from unnecessary effort; and interspersing rest periods between phases of action. However, the emphasis here is on experiencing controlled falling through voluntarily disturbing the resting body on the environment support (the bolster, a slightly mobile support system). Besides providing a different tactile environment than a bare floor, rug or foam roller, it also suspends the mover off the floor. The aim here is explicitly to stimulate sensations of fall and recovery.

Chapter 10

Vertical Dance: Re-Experiencing the World

The human body must be first understood as in interaction with its environment because it is itself the receptive matter both informed and informing.

(Sara Heinämaa 1999: 58)

As I prepare for today's performance of vertical dance at Vedauwoo, I review the choreography which has developed over the past few weeks, both inside the theatre and on the rock faces. The dance has evolved with the transition from working inside to out-of-doors, with the introduction of uneven surfaces, change in temperature and light, and we have adjusted tempos with the musicians as our movements take longer with the increased length of the rope. I am energized by the change in height where our dance takes place (50 feet above the audience as compared to 10 feet in the theatre). The rope and harness I am dancing with extends my movements in space and time to create an illusion of weightlessness and flight. These elements connect me with my movements allowing me to re-experience time, space and energy as I am dancing. I am inspired by the brilliant blue sky and cloud formations which are my 'ceiling', the impressive geologic formations which are my 'floor' and walls and the vast landscape which extends for miles in all directions. I am challenged to extend my movements and to help the audience 'see' and feel the open beauty of this environment. And yet today, the usual west-south-west wind, which has influenced the evolution of the choreography, is gusty and strong. I anticipate how this will keep me in the present, challenging me to maintain the timing, flow and freedom in my movement, but I also know it will add yet another layer to the performance as I engage with it in my dancing.

(Margaret Wilson, diary entry, 24 August 2013)

Overview

Most dance evolves in a gravity-familiar environment. This chapter describes *vertical dance*, a form emerging out of a novel relationship to gravity: airborne. The vertical dancer is suspended in the air by way of a harness around the hips. This harness is attached to a rope secured high overhead, allowing the dancer safe support to explore 360 degrees of movement space. Dancing in this airborne environment awakens somatic sensations and inspires new movement knowledge. Vertical dance provides insight into how dancer and environment collaborate in creating movement. This chapter underscores the idea that

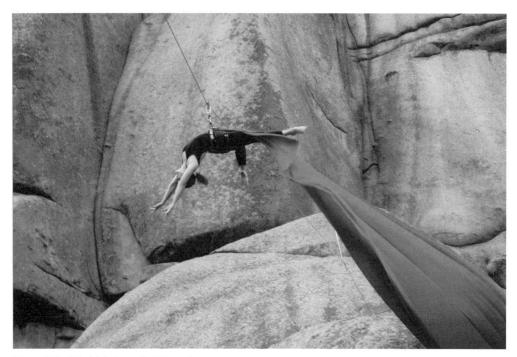

Figure 10.1: Wind (photo credit. J Harper).

regardless of where dancemaking takes place, the environment becomes embodied, shaping the dance and its meaning.

Introduction

Dancemaking implies embodying the world through movement. The phenomenon called dance emerges from a confluence of these systems within the dance context. Many processes and elements come together to shape its manner, meaning and aesthetics. While rarely brought to the level of consciousness, a complex interplay of systems dynamics are at work in the bodymind – neuromuscular, kinesthetic and cardiovascular, for example. Dancers acquire knowledge not only from experiencing these internal bodily dynamics, but also are informed by the space around them. Whether dancing in a studio, on a stage or out-of-doors, this meeting between dancer and environment is immediate, embodied and whole – a gestalt (Chow et al. 2011; Hämäläinen 2007). Here, gravity also acts as a dynamical system, shaping the dancer's movements. The dancer creates movement and meaning by exploring and exploiting the environmental kinetics (Declerck and Gapenne 2009; Damkjaer 2012). Balance, momentum, acceleration and other forces emerge from the dancer's interactions with gravity.

Vertical dance provides a fresh opportunity for meeting gravity. The engagement between dancer and environment creates new physical and mental challenges resulting in the development of new movement patterns. Such embodied knowledge carries over into other dancing contexts, as well. Here, vertical dance offers a view into how embodied cognition develops in dance specific contexts.

Affordances and ecological dynamics

A discussion of vertical dance merits introducing another perspective on embodiment – *ecological* embodiment. Moving beings and their environments are interdependent. Our soma/psyche is embodied, situated and enmeshed in whatever environments we encounter. The field of ecological psychology offers a scientific language for understanding this phenomenal interdependence. A key construct in ecological psychology is *affordance* (Gibson 1979; Turvey and Shaw 1999; Dreyfus and Dreyfus 1999; Dourish 2001; Fajen et al. 2009). Developed by ecological psychologist James Gibson in the 1970s, affordances are qualities within the environment that enable individuals to act. They are *invitations* to action (Oudejans et al. 1996; Withagen et al. 2012). As humans perceive these qualities, they enact – bring forth – possibilities for action.

Writing as early as 1966, Gibson argued that the development of knowledge and skill was not possible through mental computations and stimulus-response reactions. Perceiving is an immersive non-mediated act. Gibson coined the term 'perception-action coupling' to capture this reciprocal capability. Humans are inextricably linked by their *potential* and what the environment affords them to do (Gibson 1966). Environmental textures, structures and patterns are affordances.[1] Humans *embody* these properties to construct their location in the world and enact possibilities for action (Foster 2011; Greeno 1994);[2] all senses – smell, touch, proprioception, for example, directly transduce environmental affordances into useful, practical information.

How humans respond to the environment depends on the needs and goals of any activity. Dancemaking is a case in point. Dancers bring an abundance of embodied knowledge to any setting. The ability to interact flexibly within complex situations is a component of skill (Turvey and Shaw 1999). Dancers readily adapt to a dance studio, stage or site specific location. In each case, the moving body is the center of potential action relative to the environment (Adamson 2005). Dancers skillfully negotiate affordances – working with other bodies, thematic ideas, music or sound, props and costumes. Affordances also are specific to the task at hand and time-pressured. They change as needs change (Hirose 2002). Needs, goals and objectives often change moment by moment due to artistic, sociocultural or other concerns.[3]

This brief overview brings us to a discussion on vertical dance. Leaving the ground, the dancer is challenged to quickly adapt to novel sensations that demand a different skill set. Creating movement in the air offers a different set of affordances and calls upon the dancer to refresh familiar dance vocabulary as she meets gravity in a new way.

Vertical dance

Lawrence describes vertical dance as 'dance which takes place off the ground, against a vertical surface (commonly a wall) that becomes the dancer's "floor"…the term *vertical…* refers to the orientation of the floor, rather than the orientation of the dancer's body' (Lawrence 2010: 49).[4] My definition of vertical dance builds on Lawrence's. The dancer is suspended in the air by a harness attached to a rope. The harness acts as a conduit between the rope and the vertical dancers' body. The harness is attached to the rope, freeing the dancer from the necessity of holding her weight with her hands or arms. The harness also changes the support of the body and provides immediate information about how the airborne environment influences the dancer's movement. This support system allows the dancer to interact with a wall or other dancers in free space. The dancer is free to move in spatial directions previously unexplored. Familiar dance movements are experienced anew when the body is suspended and freed from the usual effects of gravity. At the same time, vertical dance is tremendously demanding – physiologically, neuromuscularly and perceptually. It calls upon a range of psychophysical skills in responding to novel sensory input.

The equipment and environment challenge the dancer's embodied knowledge. As a first step in vertical dance training, the dancer needs to readjust and recalibrate balance and trunk control in learning to sit upright in the harness.[5] Suspended from the ceiling, the dancer renegotiates a new frame of reference and center of mass. This balance point now is much higher than the theoretical center of gravity in the upright standing body – the attachment to the rope is through the waist loop located at the level of the navel, versus somewhat lower in the pelvis. With the base of support now higher and the limbs freed from the ground, adaptations are as much somatic as they are mechanical and neuromuscular. While dancers still experience a sense of weight, the new orientation to ground and space alters the *perception* of weight, requiring recalibration with every change of body position. This process of reorienting and recalibrating to find balance stimulates new neuromuscular patterns and control strategies.

Recalibrating spatial awareness: a new phenomenal experience

The usual way of perceiving space, and orienting in space, is based on having the feet on the ground. This is the physical experience of the body in the world (Berthoz and Petit 2008). We understand the directions up, down, forward and back relative to our earliest experiences of developing upright standing in gravity. Therefore, when the dancer has her feet on the ground, she has no need to attend to how she perceives space relative to gravity – it is part of the habitual kinesphere of engagement. However, for the vertical dancer, with her feet off the ground, suspended from the harness, sensations of gravity pass through the body in new orientations. Rotating or inverting the suspended body demands recalibrating habitual mechanical and spatial usage (Lawrence 2010; Damkjaer 2012). In a vertical environment, for example, it is possible to rotate backward from a vertical orientation 90–180 degrees or more. The dancer can also explore movement in sidelying. These options challenge the dancer's spatial familiarity of standing or lying on the ground.

The vertical dancer must hone sensory responses to the new spatial reality. In the process, the dancer must override habitual responses in the visual, auditory and proprioceptive stimuli. Inversions are particularly challenging, especially when vertical dance is practiced in a space where landmarks exist that reference up-down orientation. Here, the inverted dancer perceives the world as upside-down, and must renegotiate this optical and physical affordance. Floor becomes ceiling and ceiling becomes floor as the dancer consciously choreographs anew (Lawrence 2010; Damkjaer 2012).

Physiologically, the experience of being upside-down is very different than being upright. Our biological systems have developed to work with the pull of gravity moving through the body toward the feet (Boone and Johns 1989). Blood is pumped upward from the lower body toward the heart and flows downward from the head. In an inverted position, the normal systematic operations of the body are turned upside-down in relation to gravity. With pressure from the harness and the weight of the body, the experience of increased and blood flow to the upper part of the body is intensified. Hanging in the harness, dancers report pressure in the head and feelings of nausea that they don't experience in normal upside-down movement. The dancer is 'literally upset' (Lawrence 2010: 57), still experiencing gravity in the body, but gravity is acting on the body in a new way. As the dancer's internal environment responds to working in an inverted position, sensory information and bodily knowledge come to the forefront of the dancer's experience. The focus of attention needs to stay attuned to the immediacy of a wider panorama of freely moving variables. As the dancer practices vertical dance (with some similarity to inversions in yoga), her body adjusts to the demands of the internal and external sensory dynamics. Discomfort eases with physiological adaptation.[6] Muscular, biomechanical and motor learning adaptations also are common to negotiating a vertical environment.

Neuromuscular adaptations and motor learning

Training in vertical dance requires extensive conditioning to meet the demands of the task(s) with appropriate neuromuscular activation patterns. When the weight of the body is supported in the harness, the center of mass is redistributed around a different base of support. This provides the dancer with new information about weight and muscular effort. Dancers find themselves confronted with unfamiliar experiences that at first confuse and confound the motor system. Often, gravity can assist the movement; at other times, the pull of gravity in inversion exceeds the muscular cost demanded by upright versions of movement demands and actions.[7] For example, when the dancer is hanging upside-down, the harness induces hip flexion. The dancer must then exert extra muscular effort to extend the hips and lower limbs to maintain a straight line throughout the body, as if still standing erect. In fact, dancers discover new muscle synergies in the trunk and limbs, actively engaging these muscles strongly to keep their bodies straight while supporting their legs and low back. These patterns would not be activated in upright standing. In the position called *plank*, the dancer lies horizontally *facing* the ceiling with the body fully extended (as if lying down on the floor yet hanging in mid-air) supported only by the harness. To create a flat position in the trunk and limbs, the dancer must flex the hips and protract the shoulders sufficiently, keeping all body segments parallel to the floor to counteract the downward pull of gravity.

Other examples of inversions alter the neuromuscular control of the arms and the head. When the dancer hangs upside-down in free space, the arms 'fall' easily toward the floor. While this position simulates supporting the arms overhead in upright standing, the muscular effort required here is needed to keep the arms from flopping about. As a final example, as the dancer 'stands' with her feet on the wall and her body parallel to the floor, she faces upward rather than forward. The neck muscles co-contract much more than usual when the head is balanced on the cervical spine. This takes a lot of mental effort as well to maintain safety and stability.

Biomechanics and motor learning

Vertical dance provides biomechanical and motor learning challenges, as well. The dancer is placed in a novel learning situation that alters mechanical aspects of movement. For example, joint kinematics and force kinetics dictate movement intensity, speed, duration and many other aspects of motor control. Vertical dance places new biomechanical constraints on dancers, calling for new motor control strategies. For example, movements that require effort on the ground, such as lifting the leg above 90 degrees to the front, become effortless for the inverted vertical dancer. Rather than having to exert force to lift the leg, the dancer's leg 'falls' headward toward the ground. Muscles that act as concentric prime movers in upright gravity circumstances become eccentric controllers in controlling the leg's descent.

For the vertical dancer jumping away from the vertical wall (moving horizontally rather than vertically), airborne movements can be suspended for as long as the length of the rope will allow. The dancer is not moving against gravity, so less ground reaction force is needed to initiate the jump. At the same time, the dancer is tethered to the swing of the rope. The pendular movement of the rope affects the timing and quality of other movements in the air (Lüttringhaus 2008) – a whole new learning experience. Additionally, when landing from these jumps, only a fraction of the dancer's body weight lands on the wall ('floor'). This experience of weightlessness requires learning to grade muscle effort and joint reaction forces to land much more softly.

Vertical dance requires physically and mentally adjusting to this new world. Extensive practice is essential to build confidence and competence in the vertical dance environment. Dancers must rehearse over and over again to develop new skills of control before artistic decisions are readily available. Time is also needed to allow the motor systems to recalibrate and adapt to the challenges. While the dancer may experience less physical effort in some movements, the cognitive effort to solve the movement puzzle of the moment is not easy. Performing familiar movement in an unfamiliar orientation, the dancer develops a number of cognitive experiences and skills. The dancer must problem-solve and invent solutions to meet the demands on posture and movement. Where should the focus of attention be? Toward the floor and the acceleration of forces, or above the head where the body is oriented? Inverted actions are not always intuitive.

Meaning-making

Once the vertical dancer adapts and reorients, she dances confidently and can innovate. By this stage, the environment and the movement are one somatic whole. The dancer shifts from simply hanging from a rope to creating airborne dance. With practice, she has embodied enough facility to explore new spatial opportunities.

As in all forms of movement, the vertical dancer makes meaning in the doing (Depraz 2009). Dancers make meaning from how they are situated, sensing the body as '...a contingent project of lived and living bodies' (Ravn 2010: 30). Much of the meaning of dancemaking is grounded in physical, spatial and temporal concerns. As Merleau-Ponty has written, the body is grounded in a 'primordial...already constituted' space. In this phenomenological space we can identify with a sense of being in the world (Carman 2008: 110). The vertical dancer expands that primordial space and embodies it in training and performance.

Vertical dance extends this spatiality to bridge the 'intersection between lived space and empirical space' (Lawrence 2010: 54). This embodied experience is phenomenologically meaningful (Gallagher 2005, Parviainen 2002). As the body and the world co-create one another, they form a unique emergent relationship. The dancer moves from 'knowing' in this new spatial orientation to dancing in a vertical environment in an 'intertwining of action and awareness' (Kozel 2007: 70). She has moved from hanging from a rope, to making discoveries in an airborne environment, to dancing in the air. This is empowering. The vertical dance environment has been a proving ground for reorganization, renegotiation and affirmation of embodied knowledge.

References

Adamson, T. (2005), 'Measure for measure: The reliance of human knowledge on things of the world', *Ethics and the Environment*, 10: 2, pp. 175–94.

Berthoz, A. and Petit, J. (2008), *The Physiology and Phenomenology of Action*, Oxford, UK: Oxford University Press.

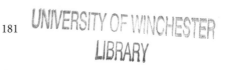

Bingham, G. (2004), 'A perceptually driven dynamical model of bimanual rhythmic movement (and phase perception),' *Ecological Psychology*, 16: 1, pp. 45–53.

Boone, T. and Johns, K. (1989), 'Cardiorespiratory and hemodynamic responses to inversion and inversion with sit-ups', *The Journal of Sports Medicine and Physical Fitness*, 29: 4, pp. 346–57.

Carman, T. (2008), *Merleau-Ponty*, London: Routledge.

Chow, J., Davids, K., Hristovski, R., Araújo, D. and Passos, P. (2011), 'Nonlinear pedagogy: Learning design for self-organizing neurobiological systems', *New Ideas in Psychology*, 29: 2, pp. 189–200.

Damjkjer, C. (2012), 'On the representation of space', in S. Ravn and L.B. Rouhiainen (eds.), *Dance Spaces, Practices of Movement*, Odense: University Press of Southern Denmark.

Davids, K. and Araújo, D. (2010), 'The concept of "Organismic Asymmetry" in sport science', *Journal of Science and Medicine in Sport*, 13, pp. 633–40.

Declerck, G. and Gapenne, O. (2009), 'Actuality and Possibility: On the complementarity of two registers in the bodily constitution of experience', *Phenomenology and the Cognitive Sciences*, 8, pp. 285–305.

Depraz, N. (2009), 'The failing of meaning: A few steps into a first-person phenomenological practice', *Journal of Consciousness Studies*, 16: 10–12, pp. 90–116.

Dourish, P. (2001), *Where the Action Is: The Foundations of Embodied Interaction*, Cambridge, MA: MIT Press.

Dreyfus, H. and Dreyfus, S. (1999), 'The challenge of Merleau-Ponty's phenomenology of embodiment for cognitive science' in G. Weiss and H. Faber (eds.), *Perspectives on Embodiment*, London: Routledge, pp 103–20.

Fajen, B., Riley, M. and Turvey, M.T. (2008), 'Information, affordances and the control of action in sport', *International Journal of Sport Psychology*, 40, pp. 79–107.

Foster, S. (2011), *Choreographing Empathy: Kinesthesia in Performance*, London/New York: Routledge.

Gallagher, S. (2005), *How the Body Shapes the Mind*, Oxford, UK: Clarendon Press.

Gibson, J. (1966), *The Senses Considered as Perceptual Systems*, Boston, MA: Houghton Mifflin.

Gibson, J. (1979), *The Ecological Approach to Visual Perception*, Boston, MA: Houghton Mifflin.

Greeno, J. (1994), 'Gibson's Affordances', *Psychological Review*, 101: 2, pp. 336–42.

Hämäläinen, S. (2007), 'The meaning of bodily knowledge in a creative dance-making process' in L. Rouhiainen (ed.), *Ways of Knowing in Dance and Art*, Finnish Academy: Theatre Academy.

Heinämaa, S. (1999), 'Merleau-Ponty's modification of phenomenology: Cognition, passion and philosophy', *Synthese*, 118: 1, pp. 49–68.

Hearn, J., Cahill, F., & Behm, D. G. (2009). 'An inverted seated posture decreases elbow flexion force and muscle activation', *European Journal of Applied Physiology*, 106: 1, pp. 139–147.

Hirose, N. (2002), 'An ecological approach to embodiment and cognition', *Cognitive Systems Research*, 3, pp. 289–99.

Kelso, J. (1995), *Dynamic Patterns: The Self-Organization of Brain and Behavior*. Cambridge, MA: MIT Press.

Kozel, S. (2007), *Closer: Performance, Technologies, Phenomenology*. Cambridge, MA: MIT Press.

Lawrence, K. (2010), 'Hanging from knowledge: Vertical dance as spatial fieldwork', *Performance Research*, 15: 4, pp. 49–58.

Luttringhaus, K. (2008), 'Alban Elved Dance Company' in J. Bernasconi and N. Smith (eds.), *Aerial Dance*, Champaign, IL: Human Kinetics, pp. 64–67.

Oudejans, R., Michaels, C., Bakker, F. and Dolne, M. (1996), 'The relevance of action in perceiving affordances: Perception of catchableness of fly balls', *Journal of Experimental Psychology-Human Perception and Performance*, 22: 4, pp. 879–91.

Parviainen, J. (2002), 'Bodily knowledge: Epistemological reflections on dance', *Dance Research Journal*, 34: 1, pp. 11–26.

Ravn, S. (2010), 'Sensing weight in movement', *Journal of Dance and Somatic* Practices, 2: 1, pp. 21–34.

Stoffregen, T., Yang, C. and Bardy, B. (2005), 'Affordance judgments and nonlocomotor body movement', *Ecological Psychology*, 17: 2, pp. 75–104.

Turvey, M. and Carello, C. (1995), 'Some dynamical themes in perception and action' in R. Port and T. Van Gelder (eds.), *Mind as Motion: Explorations in the Dynamics of Cognition*, Cambridge, MA: MIT Press, pp. 373–401.

Turvey, M. and Shaw, R. (1999), 'Ecological foundations of cognition: I. Symmetry and specificity of animal-environment systems', *Journal of Consciousness Studies*, 6: 11–12, pp. 95–110.

Varela, F., Thompson, E. and Rosch, E. (1991), *The Embodied Mind: Cognitive Science and Human Experience*, Cambridge, MA: MIT Press.

Warren, W.H. (1984), 'Perceiving affordances: Visual guidance of stair climbing', *Journal of Experimental Psychology: Human Perception and Performance*, pp. 683–703.

Wilson, M. (2013), Personal diary.

Wilson, M. and Dai, B. (2013), 'Estimating trunk compression forces in vertical dance', presentation made to the American Society of Biomechanics, Omaha, NE, September 2013.

Withagen, R., de Poel, H., Araújo, D. and Pepping, G. (2012), 'Affordances can invite behavior: Reconsidering the relationship between affordances and agency', *New Ideas in Psychology*, 30, pp. 250–58.

Notes

1 Examples of affordances are abundant in daily activities (Warren 1984; Oudejans et al. 1996). We can ascend stairs easily, not only when they are scaled to our leg length, but also readily adjust to small variations in stair height and tread. Through our experience in the world we 'measure' the width of a doorway or how far to open it, with our embodied knowledge rather than needing a yardstick. We adjust our bodily orientation as we approach the door without consciously thinking about it based on the width of our shoulders and hips, or the load we are carrying. We calibrate our positions and actions in the world based on our experience in our bodies and the environment.

2 Whereas Gibson gave primacy to vision in this perception-action relationship, Gibson's ideas have been extended by Varela, Thompson and Rosch (1999); Kelso (1995); Turvey and

Carello (1995); and Bingham (2004), who argue that we also couple with the environment through vision, touch, movement and sound; all interactions with the environment are relevant to an organism's action capacities (Kelso 1995: 189). As an emergent property of the actor/environment system, affordances provide multimodal information in real-time interaction. These temporally bounded interactions within the actor-environment system are dynamical, and meaning emerges from them (Stoffregen, Yang and Bardy 2005; Turvey and Carello 1995).

3   The reader might notice that the concept of affordances is similar to that of constraints (Chapter 3). Recently, the concept of affordance has merged with dynamic systems theory, giving rise to a new theory of ecological dynamics (Davids and Araújo 2010). Ecological dynamics enlarges the scope of affordance by focusing on the task or context in the actor/environment relationship (Chow et al. 2011).

4   In this definition, Lawrence distinguishes vertical dance practice from aerial dance. Aerial dance comes from a circus tradition that utilizes trapeze, silks and hoops – apparatus the dancer holds onto or balances on as they move in the air. Vertical dance companies and artists who work primarily with the dancer in a harness attached to a rope include *Kate Lawrence Vertical Dance* (Canaerfon, Wales), *Gravity/Levity* (England), *Il Posto Danza Verticale* (Italy), *Brenda Angiel* (Brazil), *Blue Lapis Light* and *Project Bandaloop* (US). These companies perform indoors and out of doors, both in natural and architectural locations, including in the latter, outsides of buildings, both historical and contemporary.

5   This support is unusual, and initially can cause discomfort. The leg loops of the harness create pressure on the front rim of the pelvis as well as on top of the legs, and often the back and sides of the harness place pressure on the waist.

6   The increase in cerebral blood pooling and intracranial pressure (ICP) results from an increase in hydrostatic pressure causing venous engorgement, elevated capillary pressure and filtration. See Hearn, Cahill and Behm, 2011, p. 145 for more detail on this phenomenon.

7   In the inverted cambre (hanging upside-down arching the back toward the ceiling) and high release (an upright version of the same movement), trunk-compression forces are at their highest. This is because moving the torso and head away from the vertical requires greater trunk muscle activation when the lower limbs are suspended (Wilson and Dai 2013). See also Damkjaer, 2012, p. 129.

Chapter 11

The Road Forward

In the Middle Ages, the knowledge aggregate grew at an arithmetic pace. Any learned member of society could know the bulk of extant knowledge. With globalization, the proliferation of knowledge has been exponential, boggling the imagination. It is estimated that in a mere 48 hours 'we create as much information – five billion gigabytes worth – as was created between the birth of the world and 2003' (Schmidt 2010). How can this unfathomable proliferation of information become meaningful knowledge?

This book has been an effort to ground perspectives in a developing discourse around embodied cognition in dancemaking. At this point, the *discourse* consists of topics and exchanges between somatically informed dance and embodied cognitive neuroscience. Our aim here was to track select historical developments leading to confluent dialogue and exchange. With collaborations well underway, the overarching objective was not achieving synthesis (Klein 2007), but rather, highlighting shared experiences between dancemakers and their scientific counterparts.

Current dance-science remains trans-disciplinary, practice-driven and socially networked. The exchange seeks in part to advance dancemaking *as* science (Borgdorff 2009) and science *as* 'choreographer of its own media' (Motion Bank 2009). Many issues challenge these investigations (deLahunta 2013). For one, both foresight and time are needed to integrate new knowledge and to keep the momentum going. Whether for creative ends or not, the emerging discourse hopefully will continue to thrive. Building sustainability into these shared opportunities requires vision as well as concerted effort in all phases of collaboration. This means, perhaps, developing dual and multiple competencies and 'literacies' (Harste 2003), as well as honing research designs that go beyond descriptive and prescriptive limitations. Hurdles exist. Negotiating these hurdles requires a mutual commitment to sharing information and inviting participation at many levels. Below, we've outlined some ideas to ponder as the discourse evolves.

Sustainability calls for commitment to:

1. Safeguard the holism of all participating disciplines;
2. Proceed ethically;
3. Cultivate a shared ethos of personal and professional diplomacy; and
4. Strengthen the momentum by building on initiatives already generated locally, regionally and globally.

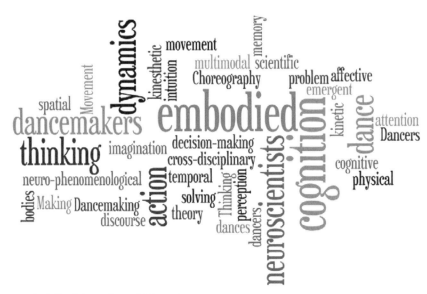

Figure 11.1: *Word Cloud:* Our call is multi-layered.

In answering the call:

1. Can we bracket[1] (suspend) our opinions, suspicions and judgments to welcome one another in dialogue? How can we recognize important differences that people bring to common goals and how can those differences impact positively on our work? How can we stay suspended in a space of understanding during times when challenging tensions arise over our differences?
2. Can we thrive in an atmosphere of reciprocity where all parties benefit? In what ways can we democratically share, create, own and disseminate our work?
3. Can we continue to evolve a non-dualist language for commerce and dissemination?
4. Can we have freer access to technologies?
5. Can we access and utilize both human and technological resources respectfully and ethically?

Recommendations forward

Below we've made recommendations for meeting this call. We steer many of these suggestions toward academic settings. Many of the challenges of feasibility and fluidity in research require access to materials common to academia, but not exclusively. Organizational designers and collaborators don't require walls. These recommendations are jumping-off points for further brainstorming.[2]

Archiving

1. Developing global Internet sites that archive materials from past research and performances (formally funded or informally produced). These can also list upcoming performances and research underway, post notices of conferences and their proceeds, lists of relevant organizations that regularly podcast talks and events, and provide interactive opportunities (blogs, etc.) for new ideas.[3]
2. Establishing separate websites for the range of published (both peer- and non-peer-reviewed) materials on embodied cognition within dancemaking. The spectrum of research could also include abstracts, commentaries, as well as personal narratives on collaborative process or actual samples of creative work.
3. Establishing a global archive of projects that will endure in time and become a historical reservoir for our work.

Networking

1. Creating global portals of visibility[3] by identifying successful partnerships and building on collaborative designs, models and research protocols.
2. Finding new ways and means of integrating non-traditional dance–neuroscience liaisons into more established settings (including, but not limited to, scientific laboratories both within[4] and outside the academy).
3. Identifying other organizations (local and global) that are catalytic to our work. For example, progressive sociocultural and business partnerships can help strengthen democratic engagement and societal interfacing. In this way, we build the trust and commitment to integration and fertilization of this unique knowledge culture, avoiding top-down and bottom-up hegemony.

Mobilizing participation

1. Recruiting a cadre of local students, laypeople and others of all ages who breathe fresh air into our endeavors and who, in turn, can benefit by participating with us.
2. Organizing seminars around topics that bring disparate areas of knowledge together with measurable objectives and mutually beneficial outcomes.[5]
3. Facilitating access to normally isolated and segregated materials, domains and technologies. For example, many kinds of institutional access exist that remain unexplored, from courtesy and affiliate faculty appointments to guest library and computing accounts. Creating new forms and capabilities that empower people by enabling access across institutions and boundaries. Opening these institutional gateways

reduces obstacles for collaboration and communication, providing better resources for creativity and innovation.[6]

Skill-building

1. Establishing cross-disciplinary trainings and other opportunities for sharing of expertise and vocabulary from each discipline – both short- and longer-term. Training also includes gaining expertise in methodologies and technologies, inventing games and other play that help explain complex concepts.
2. Creating conduits for connected learning – cross-pollinating knowledge with open-sourced arts/cultural/science clusters (organizations) that provide platforms for creativity and skill-building in new technologies and other tools.
3. Developing and disseminating syllabi and other open source materials on cognitive studies in dance.
4. Evolving accredited continuing education courses for dancemakers in neuro-phenomenology.

Advancing research

1. Promoting eco-validity in dance research.[7] Identifying feasible sites where researchers can study dance in its natural settings (physical and virtual). What scientific methodologies can best capture the choreographic process? How can choreographers contribute to the development of viable research methods without altering their ways of working? This includes mechanical factors – the type of environment, its size, location, accommodations and removal of excessive encumbrances that potentially alter or degrade the legitimacy of the project.
2. Expanding the range of topics currently in circulation by conducting new research. What other dance forms can we include and what other forms of technology are appropriate to our needs?
3. Developing models of engagement that allow for realistic time and scheduling to carry out research for all engaged parties and resources. This includes feasible designs that incorporate mutual utilization of human and material resources, such as garnering realistic time-sharing for those project managers and researchers across the various disciplines.
4. Overcoming limitations in technology and digital media,[8] by finding ways to utilize these tools within their current constraints and by asking questions that can be answered flexibly using a combination of qualitative and quantitative methods.
5. Advancing neuro-phenomenological methodology within embodied cognitive theory. To date, embodied cognition is considered a hypothesis. The hypothesis, while supported

by a number of research programs, lacks substantiation as a fully tested theory (see Shapiro 2010 for review).

Disseminating

1. Making time for reflecting on and integrating experiences in ways that all parties understand the value and impact of the results.
2. Disseminating research results in a timely manner in all the current formats, as well as inventing new ones.
3. Generating calls for proposals, abstracts, residencies and conferences whose outcomes aim to stimulate economic, as well as artistic growth.
4. Informing pedagogy[9] – supporting dance-educator consortia or other special interest groups.

Critiquing

1. What impact are these collaborations having on the development of a shared language? Does it really capture all that we are trying to say, or are we feeling minimized in the process? Language from any discourse, including dance itself, can fall short of capturing the fullness of dance experience and can be reductionist or dualist in tone. What would be the impact of 'truly overcoming the mind-body split?' (Kozel 2005).
2. How can we keep a *critique* at the core of embodied praxis?[10] If scientists are initiating the research, they should be invited and encouraged to dance, as they rarely investigate dance *as* dancers, making it difficult for them to grasp the gestalt of the experience (Blumenfeld-Jones 2009).

Sustaining and thriving

1. Determining costs, locating funders and obtaining help with managing funds.
2. Controlling costs on specific projects and obtaining help with managing of material and non-material resources. This means developing a clear sense of the ratio of resources-to-product outcomes.
3. Creating a niche for job creation in which new job roles are created and filled by dancemakers within the community.[11]
4. Integrating approaches to embodied cognition into current scholastic content as well as among community dance/health practitioners (e.g., Pilates teachers).
5. Broadening the community of interested parties who potentially can benefit. Both academic and non-academic personnel will provide portals for shared ideas. These

communities are local, regional, national or international specialists ideally committed to innovation, while respecting the ethics of intellectual property and human resources.

The current exchange is one of voracious curiosity, spirited commitment and goodwill. The dialogue remains open and agile, with many new directions for co-creating artistic performances and research. Our future and our legacy depend on honoring our mutuality and our differences as we move forward together. Our commitment to working together should not dilute the goals or processes unique to each discipline. We are poised to engage even more deeply, critique wisely and risk the unknown. As this book goes to publication, the current exchange is giving rise to many new themes that alter our premises. To this end, we invite continuing dialogue and debate.

References

Batson, G. (2012), 'Ex-scribing the choreographic mind – Dance and neuroscience in collaboration', http://seadnetwork.wordpress.com/white-paper-abstracts/. Accessed 14 September 2013.

Blumenfeld-Jones, D. (2009), 'Bodily-kinesthetic intelligence and dance education: Critique, revision, and potentials for the democratic ideal', *Journal of Aesthetic Education*, 43: 1, pp. 59–76.

Borgdorff, H. (2009), *Artistic Research Within the Fields of Science*. Bergen, NW: Bergen Academy of Art and Design.

deLahunta, S. (2013), 'Publishing choreographic ideas', in E. Boxberger and G. Wittmann (eds.), *pARTnering Documentation: Approaching Dance, Heritage, Culture*, 3rd Dance Education Biennae 2012 Frankfurt am Main, Munchen, DE: Epodium Verlag, pp. 18–25.

deLahunta, S., Barnard, P. and McGregor, W. (2009), 'Augmenting choreography: Insights and inspiration from science' in J. Butterworth, and L. Wildschut, (eds.), *Contemporary Choreography: A Critical Reader*, New York, NY: Routledge, pp. 431–48.

Depraz, N., Varela, F. and Vermersch, P. (2003), *On Becoming Aware: A Pragmatics of Experiencing*, Philadelphia, PA: John Benjamins.

Gallagher, S. and Zahavi, D. (2012), *The Phenomenological Mind*, New York, NY: Oxford University Press.

Gillespie, A. and Cornish, F. (2010), 'Intersubjectivity: Towards a dialogical analysis', *Journal for the Theory of Social Behaviour*, 40, pp. 19–46.

Harste, J.C. (2003), 'What do we mean by literacy now?', *Voices From the Middle*, 10: 3, pp. 8–12. http://www.readwritethink.org/files/resources/lesson_images/lesson1140/VM0103What. pdf. Accessed 8 August 2013.

Klein, G. (2007), 'Dance in a knowledge society' in S. Gehm, P. Husemen and K. von Wilcke (eds.), *Knowledge in Motion: Perspectives of Artistic and Scientific Research in Dance*, London, UK: Transaction Publishers, pp. 25–35.

Kozel, S. (2005), 'Connective tissue: The flesh of the network' in K. Vincs (ed.), Conference Proceedings, *Dance Rebooted: Initializing the Grid*, Ausdance National, December 2004, http://ausdance.org.au/articles/details/connective-tissue-the-flesh-of-the-network. Accessed 14 February 2013.

Linell, P. (2009), *Rethinking Language, Mind, and World Dialogically: Interactional and Contextual Theories of Human Sense-Making*, Charlotte, NC: Information Age Publishing.

Miller, E. (n.d.), 'Ecological validity', http://www.alleydog.com/glossary/definition.php?term= Ecological%20Validity. Accessed 12 February 2013.

Motion Bank Trailer (2009), http://motionbank.org/en/event/trailer-motion-bank. Accessed 22 September 2013.

Nowakowski, P., Podgorski, J.S., Pokropski, M. and Wachowshi, W. (2011), 'Interview with Shaun Gallagher Part I: From Varela to a different phenomenology', *Avant: The Journal of the Philosophical-Interdisciplinary Vanguard*, 2: 2. http://avant.edu.pl/wp-content/uploads/S-Gallagher-interview-I.pdf. Accessed 14 February 2013.

Schmidt, E. (2010), 'The Future of Google', Google Atmosphere Conference 2010, *Into the Cloud*, https://sites.google.com/site/atmospherecontent/. Accessed 14 February 2013.

Shapiro, L. (2010), *Embodied Cognition*, New York, NY: Routledge.

Vermersch, P. (2009), 'Describing the practice of introspection' in C. Petitmengin (ed.), *Ten Years of Viewing From Within: The Legacy of Francisco Varela*, Exeter, UK: Academic Press, pp. 20–57.

Notes

1   Embodied cognitive scientist/phenomenologists Shaun Gallagher and Dan Zahavi speak of the need to suspend 'realist prejudice…what appears to you is truly the state of the world… [that is more likely]…personal judgment or opinion, ego, dogma, self-interest, impulsivity and reaction' (Gallagher and Zahavi 2012: 25). The authors' concept of *bracketing* stems from Francisco Varela's first step in first-person scientific investigation: 'epoché' (Depraz, Varela and Vermersch 2003: 23).

2   Many of the ideas suggested here are also developed in a White Paper submitted to the SEAD network (Science, Engineering, Art and Design) in a call for papers (March 2012) on problems and solutions to interdisciplinarity. See Batson (2012), 'Ex-Scribing the Choroegraphic Mind – Dance & Neuroscience in Collaboration', or read other papers at http://seadnetwork.wordpress.com/white-paper-abstracts/. Suggestions for solutions to problems of arts-science interdisciplinarity can be found at http://sead.ribbot.com/.

3   This goal has been met, certainly. Three living examples at this time of publication include dance-tech.net, Marlon Barrios Solano's open-source site at http://www.dance-tech.net/, Motion Bank at http://www.motionbank.org and Irene Lapuente's multi-lingual site, 'co-creating cultures' at http://co-creating-cultures.com/cat/.

4   A case in point is Canadian dance cultural theorist Erin Manning. Manning orchestrates a 'Sense Lab' at Concordia University: http://senselab.ca/wp2/.

5   A case in point is the Watching Dance project that, among other things, serves as a resource for initiating and disseminating information on arts/dance/science conferences: http://watchingdance.ning.com/.

6   An example of institutional liaisons between science, dance and the lay public can be found in the work of the Wellcome Trust, London, UK: http://www.wellcome.ac.uk/.

7   Eco-validity is a shorthand term for ecological validity, meaning the manner and degree to which behaviors (in this case *motor* behaviors such as dance) can be observed and studied in their natural settings (Miller n.d.).

8   Digital and other technologies can limit the scope of a problem. As Shaun Gallagher notes: '…with any scientific technique you can only ask the questions that the technique allows you to answer' (Nowakowski et al. 2011: 79). A range of appropriate methodologies for research exist – self-report, observing behavior, analyzing talk, ethnographic engagement, dialogism and other forms that enable researchers to capture immediate situational utterances and transcendent phenomena (Linell 2009; Gillespie and Cornish 2011).

9   This has been an aim throughout the book, albeit indirectly stated. The Appendix is replete with explorations and multiple references to assist educators in bringing practical utility to the ideas presented. This remains a frontier for study. Special-interest groups on education are already forming, such as within Forsythe Company's Motion Bank. See Trailer Motion Bank: http://motionbank.org/en/.

10   Moving forward together ultimately means committing to building a body of valid research that evades dualist concepts of mind and body: 'To go beyond a naïve and uneducated use of introspection, and thus to enable it to become a research methodology, it seems to me that the minimum condition is first that it should be *effectively practised* by a community of researchers' (Vermersch 2009: 27).

11   I met two people in the UK whose titles were 'Director of Stuff' (a design firm) and 'Head of Discovery and Engagement' (a museum). Many new roles are possible.

Appendix I: Primer on Balance

Staying poised and upright is one of life's most striking achievements, requiring lifelong exploration and discovery (Assaiante and Amblard 1995). Relating to gravity begins at birth and continues into old age. Suspended between heaven and earth, our vertical beings are at once *geotropic* (grounded) and *heliotropic* (connected and expanding towards the sky). The conversation is mostly unconscious, involving ongoing negotiation of reflex responses and voluntary muscular tonus needed for balance control (Assaiante et al. 2005).[1] Balance is the outward expression, then, of inner problem-solving as humans encounter constant, ongoing challenges of bodily support. The bodymind is constantly negotiating three basic questions: (1) 'Where am I?'; (2) 'Where am I going?'; and (3) 'What am I going to do?'[2]

Science defines balance as a multifactorial construct (Bronstein and Pavlou 2013; Ting et al. 2009). By playing and exploring, infants develop enough postural control (PC) to maintain support in any context or task without falling (Massion 1998; Smith and Gasser 2005). An intact brain is optimal for PC and the successful execution of goal-directed movement (Assaiante et al. 2005). At the same time, the brain does not have a *control center* for balance; nor does control lie with any biological system alone. From birth, balance emerges from the interplay of biological maturation, self-regulation and experience (Thelen and Smith 1994). Babies and children learn balance first by enjoying a full spectrum of play, while risking falling. Throughout the lifespan, balance is a co-creation emerging from the flexible interplay of person, environment and task demands (Thelen 1995; Horak 2006; Duarte and Sternad 2008). At least thirteen different systems contributing to balance have been identified (Massion, Alexandrov and Frolov 2004; Krasnow, Monasterio and Chatfield 2001).

Sensory integration of somatosensory,[3] visual and vestibular input, righting- and equilibrium reflexes, the biomechanical characteristics of musculoskeletal tissues and spatial[4] and temporal values are vital ingredients. Cognitive and affective processes – perception, attention, memory and emotion – add to the complexity (Woollacott and Shumway-Cook 1990). Over the lifespan, aging processes and associated immobility, impairment, injury, habit and other factors alter responsiveness to balance challenges. Loss of balance in ageing has been associated with loss of systems complexity. With ageing (and disease) various rhythmic fluctuations in biological processes lose their temporal and spatial coherency (Manor et al. 2010; Delignieres and Torre 2009; Duarte and Sternad 2008).

Movements, emotions and thoughts disturb our balance constantly. In science, these disturbances are called *perturbations* – disturbances that challenge balance, that is, shift the body from its steady state. Common *external perturbations* include disturbances coming from the environment like descending a staircase (planned) or tripping over a crack in the sidewalk (unplanned) (Horak and Nashner 1986; Shumway-Cook and Woollacott 1995). Common internal perturbations come from our organic life (breathing, for example), from distracted attention and emotional distress. When we experience a *perturbation* that takes us off balance even slightly, the whole body reacts. These reactions are reflex patterns that help keep us from falling and stabilized over the base of support – feet in standing, pelvis in sitting, for example. Deciding to reach for a cup in a kitchen cabinet, for example, triggers a series of complex reflexes to stabilize against gravity before actually starting to reach. In this context, reaching for the cup usually is accomplished within the limits of stability. spontaneously and non-consciously. Nearly falling (stumbling, for example), or actually falling, brings balance reactions to consciousness.

Developing at birth and evolving flexibly throughout the lifespan, postural reactions are essential for orientation and navigation. These reactions are evident at birth, appearing first in the trunk (including head and neck) and developing throughout growth and development to support skilled movements (Mersmann et al. 2013; Pichierri, Murer and de Bruin 2012; Bohm et al. 2012). Postural reactions are expressed physiologically as neuromuscular 'synergies'. Synergies are global muscular patterns activated throughout the whole body in response to balance perturbations (Bernstein 1967). These neuromuscular patterns respond reflexively to right the body when falling.

Synergy patterns simplify systems complexity. They enable the nervous system to process enormous amounts of information quickly and efficiently. Synergies act quickly and globally throughout the body to restore balance. These rapid activation patterns enable us, for example, to adjust immediately to any number of different environments without conscious effort. We can readily change our walking pattern, timing or direction – even while talking on the cell phone and shopping for groceries – without falling. The same concept would apply to dancing. Dancers readily adapt to multiple environments and instructions, flexibly shaping movement vocabulary to fit new contexts (Batson 2010a).

Further, synergy patterns respond in a timely manner. Postural responses are *anticipatory* and *reactive*. In an *anticipatory* response, neuromuscular synergies activate automatically, milliseconds *before* initiating movement. Descending a staircase is a good example. The brain anticipates the descent. Synergies stabilize the body milliseconds in advance of descending. These anticipatory strategies provide the needed stability to control the falling body as it descends. Alternatively, perturbations can be unexpected (tripping, for example). These responses are *reactive*. The timing of the response may be too slow to prevent a fall.[5]

In children and adolescents, PC is far from mastered (Assaiante and Amblard 1995; Latash et al. 2005). (Note that many persons start dancing during early periods of maturation.) Synergy patterns can be elicited in infants during the first year of life, suggesting that they are to some degree innate. These synergies are not hardwired in the nervous system, however. Reflex responses may not appear readily modifiable if a fall is imminent (such as slipping on a patch of ice); such responses are not stereotyped, however. PC dynamics exhibit non-linear behavior. This implies that balance strategies are flexible, both in the brain (i.e., neuro-plastic) and in movement patterning throughout life (Woollacott and Assaiante 2002; Thelen and Smith 1994).

Balance reactions can become fixed or maladaptive for a number of reasons, however, including disease and poor postural habits. These ideally respond to re-education and training (Bronstein and Pavlou 2013). Select movement studies, such as martial arts and somatic trainings, can alter stereotypic postural responses (Pons van Dijk et al. 2013; Batson and Barker 2007; Cacciatore, Horak and Henry 2005; Ullman et al. 2010). Physical therapy fall-prevention programs also have proven effective in altering responses and reducing falls (Jacobs and Horak 2007; Rose 2011). Studies also support the effectiveness of dance for training balance in elderly populations (Ferrufino et al. 2011) and in adults with Parkinson's (Batson 2010b; Batson et al. 2013).

Attention also plays an important role in maintaining balance (Reilly et al. 2008). Since balance is dependent on the interplay of body, task and environment, the ability to selectively prioritize and allocate attention is vital to PC (Siu and Woollacott 2007). Interestingly, attending to bodily sensations can either assist or interfere with balance. Two divergent streams of thinking predominate regarding this topic (Wulf 2007; Montero 2010).[6] The question of embodied attention is particularly relevant to somatic dance trainings such as Contact Improvisation and Skinner Release – and other release techniques.

Somatic methods tend toward emphasizing attending to sensory phenomena during tasks that usually are performed more slowly than usual. Attention brings to consciousness sensations associated with patterns activated by the risk of falling (Bronstein and Pavlou 2013). For example, the Alexander Technique intervenes readily at the *anticipatory* phase of balance disturbance – in those milliseconds before the initiation of movement (or even *thinking* of initiating movement). The Feldenkrais Method® more readily attends to the phase after balance is perturbed through voluntary (Awareness Through Movement®) or receptive movement (Functional Integration®). A number of clinical studies support the effectiveness of somatic methods in improving balance. Studies on balance include the Alexander Technique (Cacciatore, Horak and Henry 2005; Cacciatore et al. 2011; Batson and Barker 2007) and the Feldenkrais Method® (e.g., Connors et al. 2010; Ullman et al. 2010; Batson and Deutsch 2004). Results from the Feldenkrais studies have garnered theoretical support from dynamical systems theory (Wildman and Stephens 2007; Buchanan and Ulrich 2003; Reese 1999; Thelen and Smith 1994). Support for the effectiveness of the Alexander Technique on balance has come from neurophysiology (Cacciatore et al. 2011).

In summary, one take-home message is that balance training should emphasize exploration, rather than rote learning. The ideal is to avoid prescriptive exercises. Rather than striving for the *right* PC strategy, people need to explore and build a flexible and adaptive postural responsiveness to variable conditions (Ting and McKay 2007) – an important message for dance educators.

References

Assaiante, C. and Amblard, B. (1995), 'An ontogenetic model for the sensorimotor organization of balance control in humans', *Human Movement Science*, 14, pp. 13–43.

Assaiante, C., Woollacott, M.H. and Amblard, B. (2000), 'Development of postural adjustment during gait initiation: Kinematic and EMG analysis', *Journal of Motor Behavior*, 32, pp. 211–26.

Assaiante, C., Mallau, S., Sebastien, V., Jover, M. and Schmitz, C. (2005), 'Development of postural control in healthy children: A functional approach', *Neural Plasticity*, 12, pp. 109–18.

Batson, G. and Deutsch, J.E. (2004), 'Effects of Feldenkrais Awareness Through Movement on balance in adults with chronic neurological deficits following stroke: A preliminary study', *Complementary Health Practice Review*, 10: 3, pp. 203–10.

Batson, G. and Barker, S. (2008), 'Effect of group-delivery of the Alexander Technique on balance in the community dwelling elderly: Preliminary findings', *Activities Adaptation and Aging*, 32, pp. 1–18.

Batson, G. (2010a), 'Understanding balance: Applying science to dance training', *The IADMS Bulletin for Teachers*, 2: 1, pp. 14–16. http://www.iadms.org. Accessed 14 February 2013.

Batson, G. (2010b), 'Feasibility of an intensive trial of modern dance for adults with Parkinson Disease', *Complementary Health Practice Review*, 15, 65–83.

Batson, G., Soriano, C., Burdette, J. et al. (2013), 'Effects of group-delivered improvisational dance on balance in adults with middle stage Parkinson Disease: A two-phase pilot with fMRI case study', *Physical and Occupational Therapy in Geriatrics* (under review).

Bernstein, N. (1967), *The Co-Ordination and Regulation of Movements*, Oxford, UK: Pergamon Press.

Bohm, S., Mersmann, F., Bierbaum, S., Dietrich, R. and Arampatzis, A. (2012), 'Cognitive demand and predictive adaptational responses in dynamic stability control', *Journal of Biomechanics*, 45: 14, pp. 2330–36.

Boisgontier, M.P., Beets, I.A., Duysens, J., Nieuwboer, A., Krampe, R.T. and Swinnen, S.P. (2013), 'Age-related differences in attentional cost associated with postural dual tasks: Increased recruitment of generic cognitive resources in older adults', *Neuroscience and Biobehavioral Reviews*, 37, pp. 1824–37.

Bronstein, A.M. and Pavlou, M. (2013), 'Balance', *Handbook of Clinical Neurology*, 110, pp. 189–208.

Buchanan, P.A. and Ulrich, B.D. (2003), 'The Feldenkrais Method: A dynamic approach to changing motor behavior', *Research Quarterly for Exercise in Sport*, 74: 2, pp. 116–23.

Cacciatore, T.W., Horak, F.B. and Henry, S.M. (2005), 'Improvement in automatic postural coordination following Alexander Technique lessons in a person with low back pain', *Physical Therapy*, 85, pp. 565–78.

Cacciatore, T.W., Gurfinkel, V.S., Horak, F.B., Cordo, P.J. and Ames, K.E. (2011), 'Increased dynamic regulation of postural tone through Alexander Technique training', *Human Movement Science*, 30: 1, pp. 74–89.

Connors, K., Galea, M., Said, C. and Remedios, L. (2010), 'Feldenkrais Method balance classes are based on principles of motor learning and postural control retraining: A qualitative study', *Physiotherapy*, 96: 4, pp. 324–36.

Delignieres, D. and Torre, K. (2009), 'Fractal dynamics of human gait: A reassessment of the 1996 data of Hausdorff et al.', *Journal of Applied Physiology*, 106, pp. 1272–79.

Duarte, M. and Sternad, D. (2008), 'Complexity of human postural control in young and older adults during prolonged standing', *Experimental Brain Research*, 191, pp. 265–76.

Feldenkrais, M. and Reese, M. (1985), *The Potent Self: A Study of Spontaneity and Compulsion*, Berkeley, CA: North Atlantic Books.

Gendlin, E. (1992), 'The wider role of bodily sense in thought and language', in M. Sheets-Johnstone (ed.), *Giving the Body its Due*, Albany, NY: State University of New York Press, pp. 192–207.

Ferrufino, F., Bril, B., Dietrich, G., Nonaka, T. and Coubard, O.A. (2011), 'Practice of contemporary dance promotes stochastic postural control in aging', *Frontiers in Human Neuroscience*, 5, pp. 169–78.

Horak, F.B. (2006), 'Postural orientation and equilibrium: What do we need to know about neural control of balance to prevent falls?', *Age Ageing*, 35: 2, pp. ii7–ii11.

Horak, F.B. and Nashner, L.M. (1986), 'Central programming of postural movements: Adaptation to altered support-surface configurations', *Journal of Neurophysiology*, 55: 6, pp. 1369–81.

Krasnow, D., Monasterio, R. and Chatfield, S.J. (2001), 'Emerging concepts of posture and alignment', *Medical Problems of Performing Artists*, 8, pp. 12–20.

Laban, R. (1980), *The Mastery of Movement*, 4th edn, London: MacDonald and Evans.

Latash, M.L., Krishnamoorthy, V.K., Scholz, J.P. and Zatsiaorsky, V.M. (2005), 'Postural synergies and their development', *Neural Plasticity*, 12: 2–3, pp. 119–30.

Jacobs, J.V. and Horak, F.B. (2007), 'Cortical control of postural responses', *Journal of Neural Transmission*, 114, pp. 1339–48.

Manor, B., Madalena, D., Hu, K. et al. (2010), 'Physiological complexity and system adaptability: Evidence from postural control dynamics of older adults', *Journal of Applied Physiology*, 109: 6, pp. 1786–91.

Massion, J. (1998), 'Postural control systems in developmental perspective', *Neuroscience and Biobehavioral Reviews*, 22, 465–72.

Massion, J., Alexandrov, A. and Frolov, A. (2004), 'Why and how are posture and movement coordinated?', *Progress in Brain Research*, 143, pp. 13–27.

Mersmann, F., Bohm, S., Bierbaum, S., Dietrich, R. and Arampatzis, A. (2013), 'Young and old adults prioritize dynamic stability control following gait perturbations when performing a concurrent cognitive task', *Gait and Posture*, 37: 3, pp. 373–7.

Montero, B. (2010), 'Does bodily awareness interfere with highly skilled movement?', *Inquiry*, 53: 2, pp. 10–22.

Pichierri, G., Murer, K. and de Bruin, E.D. (2012), 'A cognitive-motor intervention using a dance video game to enhance foot placement accuracy and gait under dual task conditions in older adults: a randomized controlled trial', *British Medical Journal Geriatrics*, 14, pp. 12–74.

Pons van Dijk, G., Lenssen, A.F., Leffers, P., Kingma, H. and Lodder, J. (2013), 'Taekwondo training improves balance in volunteers over 40', *Frontiers in Aging Neuroscience*, 5: 10. http://www.frontiersin.org/Journal/10.3389/fnagi.2013.00010/abstract. Accessed 10 October 2013.

Reed, E.S. (1996), *Encountering the World: Toward an Ecological Psychology*, New York, NY: Oxford University Press.

Reese, M. (1999), 'A dynamic systems view of the Feldenkrais Method', *Somatics Magazine/Journal of the Bodily Arts and* Sciences, 12, pp. 18–27.

Reilly, D.S., van Donkelaar, P., Saavedra, S. and Woollacott, M.H. (2008), 'Interaction between the development of postural control and the executive function of attention', *Journal of Motor Behavior*, 40: 2, pp. 90–102.

Rose, D. (2010), *Fallproof! A Comprehensive Balance and Mobility Training Program,* 2nd edn, Champaign, IL: Human Kinetics.

Shaffer, S.W. and Harrison, A.L. (2007), 'Aging of the somatosensory system: A translational perspective', *Physical Therapy*, 87: 2, pp. 193–207.

Siu, K.C., Chou, L.S., Mayr, U., Donkelaar, P. and Woollacott, M.H. (2008), 'Does inability to allocate attention contribute to balance constraints during gait in older adults?', *Journal of Gerontology A, Biological Sciences Medical Sciences*, 63: 12, pp. 1364–69.

Shumway-Cook, A. and Woollacott, M. (1995), *Motor Control: Theory and Practical Applications*, Baltimore, MD: Williams & Wilkins.

Smith, L.B. and Gasser, M. (2005), 'The development of embodied cognition: Six lessons from babies', *Artificial Life*, 11: 1–2, pp. 13–30.

Thelen, E. and Smith, L.B. (1994), *A Dynamics Systems Approach to the Development of Cognition and Action*, Cambridge, MA: Bradford Books/MIT Press.

Thelen, E. (1995), 'Motor development: A new synthesis', *American Psychologist*, 50: 2, pp. 79–95.

Ting, L.H. and McKay, J.L. (2007), 'Neuromechanics of muscle synergies for posture and movement', *Current Opinion in Neurobiology*, 17, pp. 622–28.

Ting, L.H., van Antwerp, K.W., Scrivens, J.E. et al. (2009), 'Neuromechanical tuning of nonlinear postural control dynamics', *Chaos*, 19: 2, pp. 026111.

Ullmann, G., Williams, H., Hussey, J., Durstine, J. and McClenaghan, B. (2010), 'Effects of Feldenkrais Exercises on balance, mobility, balance confidence and gait performance in community-dwelling adults age 65 and older', *Journal of Complementary and Alternative Therapies*, 16, pp. 97–105.

Wildman, F. and Stephens, J. (2007), 'Research base', Feldenkrais® Movement Institute, http://www.feldenkraisinstitute.org/articles/a_research.html. Accessed 20 January 2013.

Woollacott, M. and Shumway-Cook, A. (1990), 'Changes in postural control across the life-span: A systems approach', *Physical Therapy*, 20: 12, pp. 799–807.

Woollacott, M. and Assaiante, C. (2002), 'Developmental changes in compensatory responses to unexpected resistance of leg lift during gait initiation', *Experimental Brain Research*, 144, pp. 385–496.

Wulf, G. (2007), *Attention and Motor Learning*, Champaign, IL: Human Kinetics Press.

Notes

1   Science separates posture from movement because it associates posture with the first step in the ontological development of skilled, stabile movement (see text and references). Somatic educators see posture as a flexible continuum within movement. F.M. Alexander was allegedly the first somatic educator to equate posture with movement (Reed 1996). Moshe Feldenkrais also expounds on this in *The Potent Self: A Study of Spontaneity and Compulsion* (Feldenkrais and Reese 1985/2002) and in other works by Feldenkrais.

2   See the chart on clinical control of balance from the NeuroCom®, a division of Natus®, specialists in balance technology: http://www.resourcesonbalance.com/clinical_info/BalanceControl.aspx.

3   Somatosensory information includes sensory information arising from skin (touch or haptic information), muscles and joints (proprioception) and other tissues (fascia, etc.) (Shaffer and Harrison 2007). Although not explicitly stated in science, somatosensory input potentially includes a number of undefined, unnamed sensations associated with emotions and memories more readily acknowledged in phenomenology and psychology (e.g. Gendlin 1992).

4   The way we engage with space – how space shapes our movement – also is critical to balance, particularly for dancemakers. This topic is too large to elaborate on here. Suffice to say that humans live in a spatial sphere of worldly engagement. At once it is our habitus, a phenomenological *map* representing our body's comfort zone and a vantage point from where to begin to observe and act. This is similar to Rudolph Laban's concept of kinesphere (Laban 1980) with its dynamic tensions. Like synergies, the kinesphere is plastic as well: modifiable with experience and learning. Exploiting the range and dynamic capability of this spatial sphere is integral to dance training. Our body-in-space reciprocity is shaped by many types of experience throughout growth and development (Assaiante, Woollacott and Amblard 2000) rendering them highly variable, both between and within individuals. The variability also occurs in a moment-by-moment fashion. Put on a hat and your kinesphere adapts. Use a cell phone – same thing. Go to another terrain than your habitual home base and you find balance a little more at risk. Take up dancing and you'll definitely see your balance challenged as you work with spatial tensions.

5   The onset and pattern of recruitment of postural synergies in the trunk depends on context: where, when and in what conditions the movement is being executed. Generally, recruitment of trunk synergies should precede movement of the limbs to prepare the spine to adjust to the reactive forces from movement. For example, when a dancer prepares to tendu or perform a porte des bras, trunk muscle synergies activate milliseconds before the onset of leg advancement to maintain balance. Trunk muscles ideally activate in anticipation of the leg moving forward to prevent excessive backward movement of the trunk – a counterbalancing

reaction to limb advancement. Without this feed-forward signal to the muscles to stabilize the trunk, the dancer might readily fall during shifting weight onto the stabilizing leg. The dancer must be able to modulate the changing demands proximally (e.g., through stabilizing the head and trunk) while negotiating different motor demands peripherally in the arms and legs (Batson 2010a).

6   In addition to Gabriele Wulf's extensive support for *external* over *internal* focus of attention (2007), physical rehabilitation specialists also avoid attending to physical sensations. This perspective states that balance problems are best remediated by 'dual-task' paradigms. Dual-task protocols challenge attention and physical coordination at the same time. Dual-task suggests just that: attention is allocated between two different tasks – one cognitive and one physical – at the same time, *in real time*. A simple example is being asked to walk around an obstacle course while being asked to count backwards out loud from 100 by seven. One argument for utilizing dual-task protocols to remediate balance in the elderly is that thinking or talking out loud while walking is harder for elders to do (Boisgontier et al. 2013; Siu et al. 2008). Dual- and multi-tasking is common in dance training. Dancers are often asked to do one thing with their arms (gesture or manipulate an object, for example), while executing another complex set of steps with their legs.

Appendix II: Explorations and Reflections

Introduction

Body and Mind in Motion sheds light on embodied cognition within dancemaking by pointing to intersections between dance, Somatics and the brain sciences. The book underscores the reciprocity between thinking and moving within the context of dance praxis. A simple thought, image or idea has expressive agency; it generates movement. Movement, in turn, generates thought. The bodymind also is contextual. The brain needs a body *and* a world to create reality. Without the confluence of body and world, the brain becomes arid – bereft of the dynamic fluidity of thought.

Appendix II offers readers a range of explorations (exercises) and reflective questions designed to wed theory with practice. Whether the reader is a novice or expert, dance artist or scholar or a somatic practitioner/movement educator, the explorations attempt to ground knowledge in experiential practice.

We've designed the explorations to complement the themes in each chapter. Feel free, however, to explore any exercise at any point. Collectively, the explorations and reflections constitute simple guidelines for continuing self-investigation or discussion. We've sought to layer the experience by starting with basic awareness and build toward dance-specific skills. An exercise might begin, for example, by asking learners to orient internally, becoming present in the bodymind's readiness to move. From this somatic baseline, learners can shift toward developing their insights technically or choreographically.

The exercises emerged from our teaching over these last two years. Mostly, they have evolved in an open, uncluttered space, such as a dance studio. We encourage exploring other environments and immersive settings to bring on a whole new challenge.

Last, we include vignettes from dancers from all over the world who already have explored and written about embodied cognition in their own unique ways. Please adapt these explorations or create your own new versions. We'd enjoy hearing your feedback and learning from you.

I. Chapter 1: From Conversation to Discourse

Movement systems educator Moshe Feldenkrais is reputed to have said that a brain at rest is like thick, wet, black velvet – indicative of a silent nervous system where visual and other sensory activity are markedly decreased. Likewise, the cue 'come to quiet' in the Alexander Technique is sometimes used to quiet neural *chatter*; Alexander Technique students are trained to pause and quiet (inhibit) mental distractions before initiating movement.[1] Somatic practitioners know through experience that quieting the mind and suspending busy-ness and effort in goal-directed movement are likely to lead to improved coordination.

A. Brain on idle

Right now, simply lie on your back. Cover your eyes so that you only see darkness. Spend a good five minutes quieting your thinking. Notice all the sensory data appearing spontaneously in your brain and in your physical experience. You are not trying to track, locate or otherwise do anything but simply notice what you notice. Arriving at this state might not be as readily accessible as you intend or imagine.

Observe your brain coming to rest. How difficult is it to make this shift? What factors influence your ease and ability in coming to rest? How long does it take to reach an acceptable state of rest? Once you are resting, how do you feel as your body becomes free of distractions, preoccupations, multitasking and downright *noise*? What still pulls on your attention? How easily and quickly are you distracted? What effect(s) do distractions have on your level of tension? Are you distracted by the future (what you have to do next?) or lingering thoughts of what you were doing right before (e.g., taking dance class)? Do you have the urge to control the situation – forcing yourself to rest or otherwise interfering with the bodymind's natural processes (e.g., commanding your muscles to *soften* and *lengthen*)? See if it is possible to simply give yourself over to the experience of rest, not tracking data, manipulating your body or voluntarily altering the changing states in any way. Keep returning to the experience of simply *being*.

Reflective pause…

- How busy is your brain at rest? What is your brain doing when you are not intending to do anything?
- What neural *events* can you identify that are fleeting through your awareness? What sensory phenomena are you noticing? Photons, phosphemes or other visual phenomena (static or moving), sounds, colors, sensations of pressure or other movement forces, diffuse unnamable tensions throughout the body, temperature changes etc. What else is apparent?

- Notice how long it takes for you to quiet the noise and distractions.
- What happens when you open your eyes again? What is that transition between closing out the world and coming into the world again? How would you describe the experience? Go back and forth between quickly opening your eyes and closing them again, noticing what happens as the world disappears and reappears.
- Try this exercise several times over the course of a day – upon waking up, after shopping or tending to daily demands, after a dance class or right before bed. Note the degree to which life experience impacts on your ability to engage and disengage.

B. Stimulus detection

In the same position as you started and keeping your eyes closed, follow (track) a stimulus – a light photon or some other identifiable abstract neural event for a minute or two.

Reflective pause...

- Are you aware of changes in the flow of your weight as you track visual phenomena?
- Does the initial stimulus evolve into recognizable images, patterns, thoughts and/or feelings? Carefully note the transitions between perceiving abstract phenomena and any moment of coalescing into something recognizably meaningful.
- Given that all these neural events are *moving*, how would you describe the movement qualities?
- Do these qualities give rise to larger movement impulses?
- After exploring, record your experience by improvising or sketching and then writing your reflections to *document* the experience. What differences do you notice in the shifting states between stimulus detection and fleshing out the experience through movement and reflection?

C. Parts and wholes

Command your brain to locate a body part – e.g., simply think 'right arm', 'nose', 'stomach' etc. See what happens when the brain is given a command that is related to your own body parts.[2] Interestingly, these are not action words, but nouns; yet, the brain searches, trying to locate and clarify the meaning of the word. This sense of body ownership (one's own body parts) is a key act of embodiment. Ownership is not enough, however; the body expresses *agency*, the capacity and capability to do. Many dance scholars have drawn from phenomenology in distinguishing body ownership from agency. Cognitive neuroscientists also have researched this important distinction (see Shaun Gallagher's book, *How the Body*

Shapes the Mind (2006), for an explication of these phenomena from the perspective of embodied cognitive science).

Reflective pause...

- Notice how readily your visual attention seeks the place you have commanded. When you say 'right arm', do your eyes *target* the right arm to the exclusion of everything else? What importance does this particular penchant to mentally locate body parts have to do with dance training? How might you counter this tendency to selectively detect these stimuli and move toward perceiving the moving body as a whole?
- Identify several contexts in which sensing and locating (attending to) a body part might be useful in skilled movement coordination or where such a strategy most likely would interfere with coordination.

Toward dance praxis research

- Watch a dancer improvise a short phrase. First, have the dancer begin improvising in any way that he or she would like to do (no guidelines, instruction or agenda provided, just what arises in the moment). Then, provide an improvisational prompt of your choice, playing, for example, with the idea of shifting between two sensory polar opposites, such as lightness and darkness. What gave you the impression that the dancer was mentally working? What changes did you observe when the dancer shifted from spontaneous to guided movement intent? Make a Word Cloud[3] of the *cognitive* processes you observed.
- On a large piece of art paper, draw key elements of your own choreographic process. If you can't find continuity in your choreographic process in general, focus on a recent dance you created. With graphics and a few choice words, attempt to capture your inspiration, your process of realization, your means of working with dancers, and other elements. Compare and contrast your process to that of other dancers participating in this exploration.[4]
- To explore how sound might shape movement qualities, create a dance using only ambient sound. Then, put a piece of music to it or several different pieces. Describe how various elements are shaped in each sound context – orientation and facing, body-part usage, attention and attunements, efforts etc. For examples of a neuro-phenomenological approach to sound-shaping, see Suied, Bonneel and Viaud-Delmon (2009) and Petitmengin et al. (2009).
- In technique class, pay more attention to the moments when you are relatively still and waiting to do the next movement, rather than the movements themselves. Describe your experience in these moments: What awakens a movement impulse? What gives it

direction – somewhere to go? How readily can you let go of a movement? Can you then restore a quiet baseline of readiness?

From the dancer's vantage point

Watch the following clip to observe how a soundscape shapes a dance: http://www.watchingdance.org/news_events/rosiekaydance.php – the Sound/Music Investigation with the Rosie Kay Dance Company. This experimental work of dance was created as an exclusive collaboration between the Rosie Kay Dance Company, Emio Greco|PC and the Watching Dance Research Team. In 'Double Points' the experiment consisted of setting one movement score to different sound scores and a set amount of physical language to explore the effects of soundscapes on the perception of live dance performance. A complex dance sequence was performed to classical music, electro-acoustic music and once in silence with audible breathing patterns and footfalls. Paul Taylor's 1976 choreography 'Opus Number 64', also explored the concept of one complex dance sequence set to different sound scores (Taylor, 1976).

Alternately, silence itself can be the stimulus. In 1952, composer John Cage created 4'33", *four minutes and thirty-three seconds* of silence. The piece purports to consist of the sounds of the environment that the listeners hear while it is performed and became for Cage the epitome of his idea that any sound(s) may constitute *music* (Kostelanetz 2003: 69–70). Butoh or Mime are two examples of movement forms that explore the potency of stillness in movement. In Butoh, for example, whose ethos lies partly in the transformation of time, stillness becomes a vital counterpoint in the continuum. As Marcel Marceau states: 'To communicate through silence is a link between the thoughts of man' (Marceau n.d.).

Further reflections

Read 'Dance and Neuroscience: New Partnership' (Reynolds, Jola and Pollick 2012). Then, consider the following questions:

1. Can you think of reasons other than those stated in the article that might prompt scientists to be interested in studying dance and vice versa?
2. What sociocultural or other societal shifts are enabling novel liaisons and collaborations between dancers and (neuro)scientists?
3. Think of a specific context in making up a dance and list the cognitive processes involved. What processes, styles or ways and means render dancemaking different from didactic learning?
4. Compare your choreographic style to that of another choreographer. What are your unique organizing principles? Is there a manner of choreographing that seems alien to

you? Why? What must you do mentally and somatically to be able to choreograph under the kinds of constraints that stretch you beyond your usual pragmatic and aesthetic approach?

II. Explorations for Chapter 2 – Locating the Discourse

A. Choose a partner and decide who is partner A and who is partner B. Partner A describes to partner B what *embodiment* is, using only words, no body gestures (including facial gestures). Partner B then describes to partner A what *non-embodiment* is, but using only gestures, no words.

B. Watch one dancer make up a 10–20-second phrase in the moment. Notice your own responses to watching how the phrase unfolds and repeats. Write down whatever words come to mind to describe your experience of watching the evolution of a dance phrase. What sensations, feelings, emotions, symbols or images spontaneously arise?

   Now perform what you can remember of the phrase you witnessed without any further guidance. What happens when you actually *do* the phrase that you have witnessed repeatedly? What words can you add to your list? What is the observed dancer's response to your interpretation of their choreography?

C. Have observers sit on each side of a large, long roll of paper horizontally laid out in front of them on the floor, as if sitting at a dinner table. Have two dancers either improvise or dance a structured duet. Let the dancers on one side write a narrative *script* for the dance score using only words. On the other side, let the dancers map the choreography visually (i.e., sketch or draw what you observe).

Toward praxis research of dance and context

Since the 1970s, Contact improvisers have evolved the concept of a 'score', 'a set of perimeters within which the "dancers" interact to create and discover their "dance" ' (Nash n.d.). Like music scores, dance scores offer a structure through which to repeat, evolve and develop skill in practicing a performing art. Unlike music scores, dance-improvisation scores enable a kind of layering of experience that not only is iterative but also seeks to develop skills of perception, observation and movement (Galanter 2005). Dancemaker and multimedia artist Lisa Nelson developed the concept of 'Tuning Scores: a laboratory on composition, communication, and the sense of imagination' (Nelson 2013). Nelson's Tuning Scores evoke multisensory interaction and exploration of space, time and effort dynamics to 'provoke spontaneous compositions that make evident our opinions about space, time, action, and desire…[These improvisations] provide a framework for communication and collaboration among the players' (Nelson n.d.). Scores can emerge out of many acts. The score's framework is designed to hone both perceptual and practical skills and is rigorous research, indeed, calling upon development of multiple capabilities of observing while dancing.

Readers: Learn more about *scores* from the citations in the box below.

Burrows, J. (2006), 'Speaking dance', http://www.jonathanburrows.info/#/score/?id=3&t=content

Burrows, J. (2010), *A Choreographer's Handbook*. New York: Routledge.

Butcher, R. http://rosemarybutcher.com/

Galanter, M. (2005), *ACADEMICA*: Selected portion of Margit's MA Thesis that addressed the Tuning Score, http://tuningscoreslog.files.wordpress.com/2009/11/tuning-scores-thesis.pdf.

Nash, J. (n.d.), 'Contact Improv: A brief history', http://contactimprovla.com/?page_id=130.

Nelson, L. (2004), 'Before your eyes: Seeds of a dance practice', *Contact Quarterly*, 29: 1, pp. 20–26.

Nelson, L. (2008), 'Lisa Nelson in conversation with Lisa Nelson', *Movement Research Blog*, 1 February 2008, originally published in *Ballentanz*, April 2006 as 'Composition, Communication, and the Sense of Imagination: Lisa Nelson on her pre-technique of dance, the Tuning Scores'. http://www.movementresearch.org/criticalcorrespondence/blog/?p=2122.

Nelson, L. (2013), 'Tuning Scores Laboratory Intensive – composition, communication and the sense of imagination', workshop in Les Ailes de Bernard, France, April 2013, http://www.dance-tech.net/main/search/search?q=lisa+nelson+tuning+scores.

Stark Smith, N. (n.d.), 'The Underscore', http://nancystarksmith.com/underscore.

Stark-Smith, N. (2013), 'An emergent underscore: A conversation with Nancy Stark Smith', http://www.youtube.com/watch?v=gzG609NWp1Y.

Further reflections

1. In what way(s) does dance display 'kinetic logic'? Recall the quote from Gertrude Stein from Chapter 2. Compare it to how Maxine Sheets-Johnstone describes improvisational dance in her 2012 article, 'From movement to dance', *Phenomenology and the Cognitive Sciences*. http://link.springer.com/article/10.1007/s11097-011-9200-8#page-1.

2. According to Noland (2009), how does dancemaking pose 'puzzles for the body to solve'? Give an example. How does this kind of problem-solving differ from (or is similar to) solving a problem in mathematics?
3. Given the current interest in dance and neuroscience around embodied cognition, how can the conversation move toward an established discourse?
4. Can you imagine a shared, non-dualist language for this discourse?
5. Think of how you have described your dance process to a colleague. How might you be able to describe that same process to a scientist? As you shift this task, describe the somatic changes that also occur. How does this imagined transmission alter not only your vocabulary but also your posture, gesture, attitude etc.?
6. Think of a time when you listened to a scientific lecture and wondered what the speaker was talking about. Was there anything in the talk that was useful and practical to you? How did you mentally *map* various points to render the lecture practical or useful? How did you *make sense* of the experience, literally and figuratively?

III. Explorations for Chapter 3 – Task-Based Analysis

A. Sit at your desk with the intention to complete a short task, such as answering an email to a friend or associate you know – a fairly pedestrian answer, such as what time you are going to meet them for coffee. How does this task organize you – your thinking, your posture and gestures? What constraints keep your attention tethered to the task? How does time affect task accomplishment? Are emotional or motivational factors embedded in the task? What role do certain stylistic habits play? Now improvise the same task – compose an email on a different subject, to someone new with an unfamiliar theme.
B. Describe your anatomical constraints. Start simply – which of your legs is longer? Are your legs longer than your torso? Describe how these particular anatomical facts constrain (enhance or challenge) your skills in dancing.
C. Now list cognitive constraints – the *style* of your attention and focus, your perceptual biases, your methods of decision-making and problem solving, and your ability to remember phrases.
D. In what dance context have you recently been challenged to explore and exploit new ways of attending? Did this experience make a difference in your ability to attend in everyday life?

Place itself determines a dance outcome, perhaps even more than any other factor. Site-specific dance is a case in point. (Consult the work of multimedia choreographer/artist Stephan Koplowitz for examples of site-specific choreography: http://directory.calarts.edu/directory/stephan-koplowitz.

Set a phrase in a studio and then repeat this phrase in another location, for example in a hallway, or in a space with furniture or other obstacles. How does the place (environmental context) affect your relationship to creating the phrase now? How does the new environment affect your mood, thoughts and the resulting movements?

E. Each of the following tasks involves different layers of embodiment in the act of speaking. Describe how each of these tasks alters (challenges or otherwise affects) your performance:

- Reading aloud while sitting in a chair;
- Acting on stage with a stationary monologue;
- Acting and moving about the stage;
- Dancing rhythmically while speaking in the same rhythm; and
- Dancing rhythmically while conversing with the audience.

From the dancer's vantage point

In one sense, choreography could be defined as unique artistic outcomes arising from the strategic use of constraints. A few examples are Trisha Brown's *Accumulation* (1971) and *Watermotor* (1978), and Anne Bogart's *Viewpoints* (Bogart and Landau 2005). Look these up on YouTube and note how the constraints shaped the movement. Then, note how the choreographers, in turn, found creative ways to expand movement possibilities within the constraints. The work done with dancers of differing ability provides a glimpse into how a constraint opens up a whole world of possibilities. The seminal work done of *CANDOCO* and *AXIS dance* are good examples.

Toward dance praxis research

A. Teach an improvisational structure in which dancers can only move and gesture with the trunk, without using the arms or legs.
B. Create a phrase covering a large amount of space. Then, perform the same phrase in a much smaller space. Or, create the phrase within spherical space and then perform it in a rectangular container. Trisha Brown's early explorations were framed by the spaces she had available to her, such as the rooftop over her SoHo studio.
C. Design a task-specific experiment on embodied cognition in dancemaking that examines the effects of anatomical, temporal or special constraints on movement outcomes. Once you've identified these variables, pose a research question and outline the following:

1. What are the basic speculations or hypotheses?
2. The protocols?
3. The technologies?
4. The method of analysis?
5. Outcomes?
6. How would you disseminate results?

IV. Explorations for Chapter 4 – Reframing Embodiment

Habitual embodiment

- When next in an open area without too many obstructions (i.e., a studio), walk leisurely and pause from time to time. Do you notice whether you stop on the same foot each time you come to a pause? Does the same foot always lead and the other foot trails behind? Is your walk characterized by a habitual stopping foot and a habitual trailing foot? Why does this happen? What happens to your sense of balance if you reverse this and deliberately stop on the non-habitual foot?
- Can you notice a difference in the footfall, i.e., the quality of how each foot lands? What relationship does that have to your habitual pattern? Is there a change in breathing as you go against pattern?
- Drawing from the last exercise, can you begin to find a vocabulary for your own habit that relates to basic weight support, weight shift and balance? Where do you like to stand, face, go to next? What spaces do you avoid? Do you always 'face' a direction with the stance? Do you always transition to the next facing by the same navigating pattern?
- How do these explorations relate to your dancemaking?
- In a duet pairing, one person leads and the other follows moving side by side or one in front of the other. The leader engages in movement that is typical of their movement signature while the other follows it. Start slowly so the follower has time to engage with and understand the movement signature. After a while, see if the leader can step away and observe the partner performing the leader's signature movement. Engage in dialogue – what was it like to embody someone else's movement? What was it like to watch someone perform your own movement style? Observe another dancer going through this exercise. Reflect on what you observed of their movement journey. Did you perceive their movement quality or intensity changing when they moved through different phases of the exercise?

From the dancer's vantage point

Veteran modern dancer Deborah Hay (2012; 2013) has sought to break habitual patterns of movement as well as assumptions in her dancing. Hay describes a 'no facing' etude that she has developed over a long period of time. She had developed a 'habit' of always facing some direction when she comes in the studio, conditioned by years of assuming this postural attitude within dance. She offers insights into how to avoid 'assuming a front', in both learning movement and performance. Her demonstrations transform our idea of cardinal facing, and of conditioning ourselves to be seen in habitual ways. Try this yourself. Hay states: 'What if your choice to surrender the pattern – and it is just a pattern – of facing a single direction or fixing on a singularly coherent idea, feeling, or object when you are dancing is a way of remembering to see where you are in order to surrender where you are' (2012).

The language of embodiment

In *The Six Questions*, dancer/author Daniel Nagrin prescribes exercises for exploring the interrelationship between words and movement (Nagrin 1997). Here, we create our own exercises to uncover embodied experience and verbal articulation.

- Improvise in the studio on the topic of embodiment. How do you demonstrate that concept in movement and how does embodiment manifest in your movements? Reflect on how pedestrian or habitual movements transform with deeper states of embodiment. Focusing on them now, how would you describe the feeling of revisiting the movement with this awareness? Share these experiences and reflections with other dancers. What distinguishes your approach to embodiment from someone else's?
- Teach a 10–20-second phrase to a class only using words. The teacher uses his/her voice as if speaking everyday prose – simple narrative. No gesturing with arms, trunk or face. See how successful you are in getting your ideas across. Do this for different types of phrases – classical ballet style, release-based, jazz or ethnic. Compare notes on what is different about learning by way of movement demonstration vs. words. What are the means through which dance so readily communicates? What do words add that helps dancers achieve the meaning? In what ways are words useful in learning dance at any stage? How and at what stages can they hinder learning?
- Take an abstract paragraph from a textbook, in mathematics or political theory, for example. Avoid texts that are of the 'how to' order (such as 'car maintenance'). Speak the words and have your dancers improvise on the text. Divide the dancers into trios and have each trio select from their movements to create a short dance (1 minute). Compare the outcome.
- In *The Meaning of the Body* (2008), Mark Johnson argues that our understanding of the world comes from our experience in the world. Using verticality as a 'schema', our general understanding of an idea is based in our embodied experience. For example, up is a direction away from the ground, and correlates to levity, hope, aspiration etc. Understanding the term 'I am feeling up today' comes from our

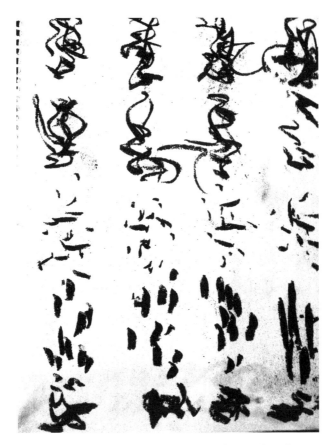

Figure II.1: Batson's improvisational 'glyph' (*Meta-academy* 2014, www.dance-tech.com).

physical experience of moving in an upward direction. Explore through movement two opposing dimensions (up or down, for example). Now try contrasting your movement with the word. For example, think of bursting with joy, but move and gesture as in retreat. Test this on yourself, or observe a group of dancers performing either complementary or polarized directional words. Reflect and record your impressions.

- Contact Improvisation pioneer Nancy Stark Smith offers an interesting way to dialogue between brain and movement in a process she calls 'the hieroglyphs' (see Figure II.1). This process provided Nancy with one inroad to clarifying the transition between dancing and writing. Here, content was less important than process – catching the immediacy of flow of thought with movement and being able to translate that onto paper. You can try out this process of 'glyph' writing by reading Nancy's article (1982).

Further reflections

1. Dance has been described as *embodied knowing*. How is *knowing* in dance different from other ways of knowing?
2. Provide a definition of embodied knowledge by giving examples in your own dance experience (practice, choreography, pedagogy). How (and in what ways) is embodied knowledge in dance different from that of acting, sports, martial arts or other mindful/somatic practices?
3. What are embodied first-person methodologies? Provide examples of research across arts, sciences and humanities.
4. Think of two choreographers whose work is diametrically opposed in terms of their somatic/conceptual embodiment. Describe the differences. Why would both approaches be considered embodied?
5. In 1957, Paul Taylor performed 'Duet', a dance where he stood still for four minutes from the point where the curtain opened until it closed. How does this piece speak to embodiment? How have you deliberately choreographed a piece either augmenting or diminishing qualities of embodiment? What impact did this have on the audience?

V. Explorations for Chapter 5 – Enaction

Brain on- and offline

In the Constructive Rest Position (CRP),[5] close your eyes and become aware of all the sensations – the proprioceptive sensations inside and on the surface of your body, and the more kinesthetic sensations that arise with surface contact of body-to-space. Begin to enliven your *exteroceptive* senses by kinesthetically sensing the environment. What sensations call you most? Track your transitions from sensing your inner world to perceiving the outer world. Describe your *style* of transitioning – the intensity, pace, effort factors and other features. Consider your *style* of enaction: In perceiving kinesthetically, are you more *receptive* (awaiting the arrival of a stimulus) or *active* (searching for and directing stimuli)? Perhaps your style changes with context. How do your preferences for this type of kinesthetic bonding relate to the way you learn movement material?

Kinesthetic Empathy

Dance researcher Ivar Hagendoorn (www.ivarhagendoorn.com) notes that people who are watching dance (spectators, viewers, audience) 'internally simulate' movement sensations of 'speed, effort, and changing body configuration' (Hagendoorn 2004).

Through watching alone, we can begin to understand the mover's intentions and 'map' the qualities of their movement onto our own – acting at a deeper level of embodiment and engagement – as if we, ourselves, were the 'actors' in the situation. This phenomenon of kinesthetic empathy is well known among dancers and integral to the process of communicating dance.

Look at the Mind Map on the Watching Dance website.[6] Here, a consortium of researchers in kinesthetic empathy has been investigating audience responses to observing dance. Answer the two questions below:

1. Look under the different 'pleasures' of the Map – visual, interpretive, kinesthetic, musical and emotional. Drawing from two of the different pleasures of your choice, comment on your experience of watching a recent dance performance. For example, (guidelines only):

    -   How did those particular pleasures help you 'make sense' of what you saw?
    -   Which of the pleasures make watching that particular dance captivating and interesting?
    -   What bodily feelings and emotions emerged from seeing the dance?

2. Did the Map help you grasp the complexity of kinesthetic empathy? How?

From the dancer's vantage point

Compare and contrast the choreographic empathy in the early work of Martha Graham (early modern dance) to that of early postmodernists and modern dance 'leftovers'[7] David Gordon and Valda Setterfield or Trisha Brown. Repeat this exercise drawing from the work of more contemporary dancemakers.

Learn more about kinesthetic empathy, or simply refresh your understanding by reading the scholarship. Read the book, *Rhythmic Subjects: Uses of Energy in the Dances of Mary Wigman, Martha Graham and Merce Cunningham* (Reynolds 2007) on the different manifestations of Kinesthetic Empathy among these choreographers. Read, as well, *Choreographing Empathy: Kinesthesia in Performance,* by Susan Leigh Foster (2010). Both books are excellent sources on kinesthetic empathy in dance aesthetics and performance.

VI. Explorations for Chapter 6 – Attention and Effort

Styles of attention

A. List as many synonyms as you can for the word *attention*. Compare your list with these words from the thesaurus: key, center, crux, feature, highlight, spotlight, awareness, recognition, care, carefulness, cognizance, consideration, heed, intimacy, knowledge, mark, note, notice, observe, perceive, regard, remark, sense. How do these different words expand your ideas about what attention is and how it functions?

B. How would you describe your own habit(s) in regard to perception and attention? Do you tend toward a narrow focus – exacting in the way you look at details? Is this related to visual acuity (nearsightedness, for example?) Or, have people described you as 'spacey'? On a spectrum of pinpointed to expansive gaze, where is your tendency? How readily can you shift between styles of attention? After spending 15–20 minutes on the phone (narrow and contracted focus), do you deliberately recuperate by allowing your focus to open and widen?

C. How often do you experience states of attentional *flow* (Cziksentmihalyi's 1990 model of absorption and immersion in a task)? In what context(s)? What dance experience(s) provided a feeling of effortlessness? Why? Which experiences were unduly effortful? Why? What other factors might contribute to your feelings of effort versus those of effortlessness?

Toward dance praxis research

- What is unique about dance is that the point of attention is dynamic – changing, rarely fixed and pregnant with stylistic possibilities. Play with the notion of contrasting a wide panoramic focus with a narrow one. Choreograph a 15–20-second movement phrase and memorize it enough to repeat easily. Perform it as you ordinarily might for your *pilot* audience (a group of students, for example). Then, change the focus to a narrow/objective focus as if you are talking on your phone. Then, perform the phrase from a wide/subjective focus, as if you were skydiving.
- Create a short movement phrase for your partner. Teach it to them first using a cue that indicates an internal focus of attention ('Think of your feet'). Have them perform the phrase for you while utilizing an external focus of attention ('Pay attention to the way your body connects to space'). Compare the differences. How easily did the partner learn the phrase? What effect did each prompt have on realizing the movement goals?
- Perform a phrase you know from a class, or a section from a set choreography. As you perform this sequence, mentally or verbally cue the direction or intention. Consciously notice just how you cue your body to move. These can be as specific as 'feel the legs connect to the floor' or 'lead with the pelvis', or qualitative, such as 'let the arms float'. Does awareness of the body part while performing the sequence change your experience? In what way(s)?
- Mirrors: how does dancing while facing a mirror direct your attention? How does this change when facing away from the mirror? What information do you attend to in either situation? What information do you need to filter out?

From the dancer's vantage point

A. Ballet Frankfurt choreographer William Forsythe asked the dancers to perform as if they were always aware of something behind them. You can read more about this verbal prompt and others Forsythe uses for focusing attention in Caspersen (2011).

B. Read the article from *Journal of Dance Education* by Brodie and Lobel (2008). There are some wonderful exercises on perception that you can try here. An alternative read is Irene Dowd's *Taking Root to Fly* (1995), both an artistic and personal rendering of her teaching through the lens of Ideokinesis.

C. Notice the orientation, attention and attunement in the 2004 YouTube clip of the Paralympic dance troupe Thousand-Hand Guanyin. All 21 of the dancers have been deaf and without speech since birth. Relying only on clapping signals from trainers at the four corners of the stage, these extraordinary dancers deliver a visual spectacle of dual attention: http://www.youtube.com/embed/7vs-H7xLnrs?rel=0.

Further reflections...

1. What methods are emerging for training attention within dance?
2. What are the markers of success of these methods?
3. How can we identify problems of attention control in dancers?
4. List characteristics of embodied attention. What difference does it make for the emergent qualities within the dance?
5. Give an example of an approach to practice that would help dancers who are easily distracted. How would you train dancers to sustain an active, lively and flexible focus while dancing? How readily can you employ these training methods on the spot (in the classroom or rehearsal)? What other methods have you learned outside of dance that have helped you?

VII. Chapter 7: Training Attention – The Somatic Learning Environment

In the following exercise, stay open and curious in your movement investigations. Don't try to do anything *right* or *correct yourself when you think the movement wasn't what you intended.* Allow yourself to move without being tied to a sense of achievement. Try not to impose any aesthetic (technical, choreographic or performative) on your exploration. Allow yourself to come from a place free of any specific form of movement vocabulary. If you are stuck for what to do next, wait in *open attention*,[8] when nothing appears to be happening (i.e., without engaging in motor processes of doing). Wait for the next impulse to arise. To quote UK dancer Gill Clarke, '[A]n effort made consciously to control the outcome... usually ends up derailing the activation' (Clarke, Cramer and Müller 2010: 212).

A. In an open space or studio, walk at a comfortable pace in any direction. From time to time, give yourself the command to stop and rest for at least 20–30 seconds. Really rest – do nothing; empty your mind of thoughts. Then, go again. Spend a good 5–10 minutes at this exercise.

B. Close your eyes and visualize where you are and the layout of the room. From what vantage point do you see yourself in the room? See all its architectural features distinctly as you can. Now visualize yourself improvising in that space. How do you start? What begins to shape the movement?

C. With eyes open, explore improvising to the four corners – north, south, east and west. As you come to a resting pause between changing directions, be aware of orienting to that specific direction. Once you've arrived at a new orientation, now come to full rest.

D. In the Constructive Rest Position, come to a quiet state and decide to open your right knee to the side – one arcing motion of your thigh to open and return your leg to standing. Do this action only one time. Take at least two minutes to track the movement feedback after performing it once. Now come to standing, still staying in the realm of ease and calm. Notice the differences between the two sides of the body.

E. Have a partner choreograph a challenging phrase for you to learn. The phrase can be about 10–20 seconds long. It should contain those elements that you find difficult to accomplish – effort dynamics, timing, level changes, body-part use and transitions, etc. Explain to your partner some of these challenges to help guide the choreography:

   • Have the partner show you the phrase once.
   • Perform the phrase as best as you can full out without any marking or other preparatory practice.
   • Lie down and rest fully for about two minutes.
   • Rise and perform the phrase again. Note whether the rest was helpful in performing the phrase the second time.

Further reflections...

1. What environment, context or state best affords the brain a state of rest?
2. What are the benefits of allowing the brain to *go offline*, to rest and not attend to anything deliberate? For example, sleep is associated with the brain at rest. Often, however, the brain is not *resting* but actually continues to process the day's activities during sleep. Various sleep states (including dream states) are not a form of *rest* but vital processes of learning and memory consolidation and integration.
3. How would you describe resting states that the brain needs during waking hours? Do you rest during the day? Describe your practices – what places, postures and actions are involved? For how long do you rest?

4. Think of how rest is used in somatically informed dance or other somatic practices? What are these states? How do you achieve them? Provide examples of your own experience both inside and outside of dance.

5. Read the 2010 article on intentional rest by Batson, *Journal of Dance and Somatic Practices*.

VIII. Explorations for Chapter 8 – The Mental Practice of Motor Imagery

Clearly picture yourself *running* in some context. Now, simultaneously say out loud the word *throwing*. You will readily see how imagery can be strongly motoric, priming that movement and only that movement. Mental practice of motor imagery offers a rich archive of exercises and explorations from many different dance artists and educators. At the same time, there is still a great deal to learn about the differences between different types of imagery – visual, kinesthetic, auditory – and their effects on movement creation.

Visual and tactile-kinesthetic imagery as prompts for improvisation

Teach a class in improvisation using visuo-spatial imagery as a prompt to create movement. For example, explore different imaginary vectors transecting the body or space. Take at least 20–30 minutes to explore how envisioning this particular visuo-motor image influences movement choices. Choose a variety of visual images from art that express some common theme, such as a dynamic spiral or other dynamic shape with communicative power.

Pause…

Change the prompt to a tactile-kinesthetic image. You might, for example, use skin as a prompt, its contact with the floor, the air or with other dancers. Move with eyes closed and eyes open. Use fabrics, textures or surfaces to gain a basic context for the feeling of bodily contact as the starting point. Take the same amount of time to explore how a more tactile-kinesthetic prompt influences movement choices. Reflect with your dancers on the differences in experience and outcome. What important roles do these different modes of imagery play in your processes of discovery, creation and performance? How does each imagery modality affect the process of creating movement? Which images were the most generative – which afforded the most accessibility, automaticity, vividness and clarity, flexibility of usage? As a teacher, did you gain insight into the use of language and movement creation for teaching or performance? Describe how each mode facilitates:

- The generative power to move
- Ease of movement creation
- Vividness and clarity of the movement conception
- Transitional capability
- Full use of inner-body space
- Connectedness of the whole body
- Other differences

IX. Explorations for Chapter 10 – Vertical Dance

This chapter introduced vertical dance as an example of how the environment impacts on the body in the creation of new movement. The novel relationship afforded by this experience allows dancers to reconfigure the way gravity works on the body. When the relationship to gravity changes in such a profound way, we are presented with the opportunity to revisit and relearn new skills. Other movement forms such as yoga, contact improvisation and many somatic techniques offer some similar opportunities for discovery. Yet, the unique natural environments afforded vertical dance and their level of risk makes a difference, certainly.

Further reflections…

1. Considering the enaction theory, how does vertical dance enhance the capabilities of our sensemaking physiological body?
2. How does the environmental context influence posture and movement choices?
3. How does moving in this novel context influence our perception in the world?

Basic orientation to gravity – upright standing

Our orientation in the world can come from two sources – internal and external. Internal direction is called *egocentric*, and it means that we orient from where we are in relation to the space, whereas *allocentric* would be to orient from the cardinal directions.

Baseline *egocentric* orientation: stand in a natural setting and look out from your eyes at the visual shape of an 'oval' in front of you. Sense the roundness of your eyes and how they are resting in their skeletal eye orbits. What do you actually see from this vantage point of near-self? Notice that you are enmeshed in a sphere. How much space is above you, below you and to the sides of your head? Begin moving throughout the studio space. Notice how easily you balance the head, neck and trunk as you move through space. How do these body parts help you navigate and orient in the space? How does gravity influence the action of moving the limbs? Imagine doing the same exercise in a different relationship to gravity – how heavy are your limbs when you are lying on the floor? How do you sense the weight of your head in a handstand or yoga inversion?

Baseline *allocentric*: specificity of location carries historical and functional impact on both the dance and the audience. Note the impact of 'upstage' and 'downstage' on dance, dancers and audience, e.g. Compare your sense of orientation from the view of the stage vs. the view from the audience.

Wayfinding – steering and navigating

Orienting is also an intentional way of moving through space. As an exercise, you can play with orienting, starting in restful standing and moving through space in the following ways:

- Navigating from here to there.
- Landing, taking leave, path creating – distinguish between each of these.
- Grounding the navigation in one somatic system (e.g., organs as 'compass').
- Using external landmarks to organize and coordination movement.

For example:

A. Move in response to a bodily cue, such as 'follow the breath', 'sense how sound influences the weight of your limb' or 'follow light with different body parts'.
B. Moving through the space, again, notice what happens in your body when you change direction. What body parts lead or follow – experiment with your vision or focus instigating the change. What happens when you change directions by initiating the movement from the rib cage or pelvis? What do you notice in these explorations about your decision to change direction – what affords a new orientation? Periodically close your eyes without stopping your movement. Go between states of open visual awareness and closed awareness sensing your relationship to the environment – physical, sensorial and intentional.
C. Steer through the space from your feet. Then, let yourself be led by other body parts – knees, pelvis, ribs, heart and head. Note differences in flexibility and ease of navigation. These differences can surface particularly when changing directions at right angles vs. exploring curves in space.
D. Orient and steer within the space by leading with the central apex of each spinal curve – e.g., T1, T12, L3, S2 (internal source of orientation). Allow the spine to shape to specific objects in the space –chairs, cubes, corners, surfaces, light fixtures or light spaces.[9]
E. Steer by way of the ecology of the space –floor patterns, light or sound sources, color etc. Improvise with sound cues. Reflect on the differences and similarities in these three experiences.
F. In a relatively unobstructed room (or studio) face south. Stand quietly, eyes closed. Notice the light in the room. Listen to the ambient sounds in the room – notice how you attend as you search for sound and how your experience changes as you locate the

sound(s) and continue to listen to them. How do these sounds shape your thoughts, feelings and sense of inner movement? (Note: you can also do this with breath or light or other phenomena, obviously.) Notice the sounds coming from inside and outside your body. Notice how you are oriented. How confident do you feel in space? With eyes closed, change directions (e.g., to the east or west). Cover the four corners in this exercise before you open your eyes.

Toward dance praxis research

- In technique class, pay particular attention to how sound organizes the class – the music, the teacher's cues, the movement dynamics, as well as how it organizes you. If possible, consciously choose a different part of the room midway through class. How do the sights, sounds and your perceptions change?
- Compare your experience in A (above) by allowing the choreography to be shaped by the sound surround of birdsong outdoors. Repeat the exercise in different seasons.
- Choreograph a short phrase while standing. Repeat the phrase in a different orientation to gravity, perhaps at a low level and prone orientation or transforming all of the movements into jumps.

From the dancer's vantage point

A. Watch 'Roped Together' by Kate Lawrence. This performance was inspired by the camaraderie that mountain climbers have for each other. How does the choreographer use the vertical space and the dynamics to create an experience of fear, tenderness and weightlessness in this environment? See http://www.youtube.com/watch?v=-4FQ-Qvq_FY.

B. In 'Exuvia', choreographed by Wanda Moretti of Il Posto Danze Verticale, how does your experience watching the dancers change throughout the piece? Notice how time and effort become exaggerated in this duet that takes place on the outside wall of the building: http://www.youtube.com/watch?v=rKVhicFH2nk.

Further reflections…

1. What effect does orienting have on how we initiate movement?
2. How would you describe some of the differential effects of gravity when standing on your hands, working with inverted postures, lying on the floor or partnering?
3. When viewing movement from different spatial vantage points, do you experience physical sensations of that particular orientation?
4. How can we build more novelty into teaching and skill building in movement by using different environments?

References

Batson, G. (2010), 'The Somatic practice of intentional rest in dance education – Preliminary steps towards a method of study', *Journal of Dance and Somatic Practices*, 1: 2, pp. 177–97.

Bogart, A. and Landau, T. (2005), *The Viewpoints Book: A Practical Guide to Viewpoints and Composition*, New York: Theatre Communications Group.

Brodie, J.A. and Lobel, E.L. (2008), 'More than just a mirror image: The visual system and other modes of learning and performing dance', *Journal of Dance Education*, 8: 1, pp. 23–31.

Brown, T. (1971), 'Accumulation,' *Trisha Brown Dance Company Repertory*, http://www .trishabrowncompany.org/?page=view&nr=264#main. Accessed 6 April 2014.

Brown, T. (1978), 'Watermotor,' *Trisha Brown Dance Company Repertory*, http://www .trishabrowncompany.org/?page=view&nr=975. Accessed 6 April 2014.

Cage, J. (1952), The premiere of the three-movement *4'3"* was given by David Tudor on 29 August 1952 at Woodstock, New York.

Caspersen, D. (2011), 'Decreation: Fragmentation and unity', in S. Spier (ed.), *William Forsythe and the Practice of Choreography: It Starts From Any Point*, London: Routledge, pp. 93–100.

Clarke, G., Cramer, F. and Müller, G. (2010), 'Minding motion' in I. Diehl and F. Lampert (eds.), *Dance Techniques 2010*, Leipzig: Henschel Verlag, pp. 199–229.

Cszikszentmihalyi, M. (1990), *Flow: The Psychology of Optimal Experience*, New York: HarperCollins.

deLahunta, S., Clarke, G. and Barnard, P. (2009), 'A conversation about choreographic thinking tools', *Journal of Dance and Somatic Practices*, 3: 1–2, pp. 243–59.

Dowd, I. (1995), *Taking Root to Fly*, Northampton, MA: Contact Editions.

Foster, S.L. (2010), *Choreographing Empathy: Kinesthesia in Performance*, New York: Routledge.

Hay, D. (2012), 'I think not', 24 April 2012, http://hztfestival.wordpress.com/tag/deborah-hay. Accessed 7 October 2013.

Hay, D. (2013), interview, *Hay's Days: A Deborah Hay Celebration*, http://www.youtube.com/ watch?v=P7YjyNofrC0. Accessed 7 October 2013.

Johnson, M. (2008), *The Meaning of the Body*, Chicago: University of Chicago Press.

Kostelanetz, R. (2003), *Conversing with Cage*, London, UK: Routledge.

Marceau, M. (n.d.), http://www.thinkexist.com. Accessed 15 February 2013.

Nagrin, D. (1997), *Six Questions: Acting Technique for Dance*, Pittsburgh: University of Pittsburgh Press.

Nash, J. (n.d.), 'Contact Improv: A brief history', *Contact Improv LA, Contact Improvisation in Los Angeles*, http://contactimprovla.com/?page_id=130, Accessed 5 March, 2014.

Noland, C. (2009), *Agency and Embodiment: Performing Gestures/Producing Culture*, Cambridge, MA: Harvard University Press.

Petitmengin, C. (2007), 'Towards the source of thoughts: The gestural and transmodal dimension of lived experience', *Journal of Consciousness Studies*, 14: 3, pp. 54–82.

Reynolds, D. (2007), *Rhythmic Subjects: Uses of Energy in the Dances of Mary Wigman, Martha Graham and Merce Cunningham*, Binsted, UK: Dance Books.

Reynolds, D., Jola, C. and Pollick, F.E. (2012), 'Editorial introduction & abstracts: Dance and neuroscience – New partnerships', *Dance Research*, 29, pp. 260–69.

Stark Smith, N. (1982), 'Dance in translation: The hieroglyphs', *Contact Quarterly*, 7: 2, pp. 43–46.

Suied, C., Bonneel, N. and Viaud-Delmon, D. (2009), 'Integration of auditory and visual information in the recognition of realistic objects', *Experimental Brain Research*, 194: 1, pp. 91–102.

Sweigard, L. (1974), *Human Movement Potential: Its Ideokinetic Facilitation*, New York: Harper & Row.

Taylor, P. (1957), 'Duet', in *About Paul Taylor*, American Masters website, http://www.pbs.org/wnet/americanmasters/episodes/paul-taylor/about-paul-taylor/719/. Accessed 14 February 2013.

Taylor, P. (1976), 'Opus Number: 64', *Paul Taylor & Dance Company*, 'http://ptdc.org/repertoire/polaris/. Accessed 6 April 2014.

Vineyard, M. (2007), *How You Stand, How You Move, How You Live: Learning the Alexander Technique to Explore Your Mind-Body Connection and Achieve Self-Mastery*, New York: Marlowe & Company.

Notes

1   Both of these examples come from Batson's personal experience in somatic education classes. They have entered into a common somatic lexicon and cannot be traced back to their original sources.

2   Credit for this exercise goes to Missy Vineyard, Alexander Technique teacher, who presented a workshop on thinking at the 2008 Alexander Technique Congress in Lugano, Switzerland. See also, Vineyard (2007).

3   Instructions for making a Word Cloud can be found at www.wordle.net. See Figure 6.1 as an example. Mind-mapping is another option. You can find instructional guidelines in Chapter 1, footnote 1.

4   Readers can read about the complex challenges in the collaborative efforts of a cognitive scientist and two dance researchers in developing a 'process model' of a 'choreographic thinking tool' (deLahunta, Clarke and Barnard 2009: 51).

5   The *Constructive Rest Position* was developed by Dr. Lulu Sweigard (1974), a pioneer in Ideokinesis. The CRP also is called semi-supine in Alexander Technique. The position places bodily joints in neutral and allows gravity to act on the body horizontally and with reduced force. Lying on the floor with the legs bent to 90 degrees, the spine in neutral, the head flat on the floor, or supported by a small towel, and the arms crossed over the chest.

6   http://www.watchingdance.org/research/kinesthetic_empathy/index.php. You can find and explore this Mind Map using the left-hand navigation bar on this page or click on http://www.watchingdance.org/Mind_Map/Interactivemindmap/index.html.

7   Attributed to David Gordon in the video, 'Making Dances: Seven Post-Modern Choreographers'. Video trailer available at http://www.youtube.com/watch?v=IHtSUQ-3FnI.

8   My knowledge of this term is that it is attributed to Emilie Conrad as a vital process in teaching Continuum Movement – a space where attention acts as a listener or witness to all that has been stirred up in sound and movement: http://www.continuummovement.com.

9   Credit goes to Irene Dowd for first introducing Batson to the concept of leading with various spinal segments in movement in 1977. Dowd would have movers imagine an 'eyeball' on these various segments to focus awareness on a body part that might not readily be accessible.

Index